FOOL
BRITANNIA

FOOL
BRITANNIA

*Headline-Making Stories
from Jobsworth Britain*

by

Sue Blackhall

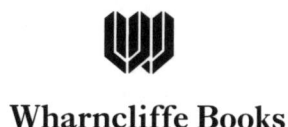

Wharncliffe Books

First published in Great Britain in 2010 by
Wharncliffe Books
an imprint of
Pen & Sword Books Ltd
47 Church Street
Barnsley
South Yorkshire
S70 2AS

ISBN 978 1 84563 117 8

A CIP catalogue record for this book is
available from the British Library.

Typeset in Palatino by
Phoenix Typesetting, Auldgirth, Dumfriesshire

Printed and bound in England by
CPI UK

Pen & Sword Books Ltd incorporates the imprints of Pen & Sword Aviation,
Pen & Sword Maritime, Pen & Sword Military, Wharncliffe Local History,
Pen & Sword Select, Pen & Sword Military Classics, Leo Cooper,
Remember When, Seaforth Publishing and Frontline Publishing.

For a complete list of Pen & Sword titles please contact
PEN & SWORD BOOKS LIMITED
47 Church Street, Barnsley, South Yorkshire, S70 2AS, England
E-mail: enquiries@pen-and-sword.co.uk
Website: www.pen-and-sword.co.uk

Contents

Introduction

We in Great Britain are now living in not so much a Nanny State but a very strict Governess one with the powers that be wielding a very big cane if we fall foul of the 'rules'. We are disciplined, indoctrinated and very often derided, for just wanting to carry on our ordinary, everyday lives.

Motorists are made out to be monsters, hell-bent on causing mayhem on our roads by recklessly blowing their noses, laughing or munching on a snack as they sit behind the wheel.

Over-pedantic 'Health and Safety' officials are banning every-thing that has quite happily (and safely) been a part of life in days long past such as traditional playground games, bonfires (preferring 'virtual reality' ones), real Christmas trees, reindeers walking on snow, bunting, doormats, paddling pools and popping pebbles in streams.

Shoppers are being banned from our supermarkets for not smelling right or entering with a balloon in their hands. And now you need ID to prove your age when buying anything from a slice of quiche to a greetings card depicting bottles of wine. There was also the incident of the little boy barred from buying wine gums because he was too young to be making an alcoholic purchase.

In short, the term 'political correctness', far from being applied to ensure sensible precautions or a sense of fair play, is more often than not alluding to stringent, inexplicable stupidity. Common sense does not prevail. Sometimes it doesn't even get a look in.

Jokes that would once have been simply dismissed as funny are now being branded 'racist' or 'sexist' or 'offensive' – so too is any entertainment which might contain an element that does not conform to today's politically correct enforcement. Who could ever have thought that music hall star Al Jolson would have to 'change colour' in the re-telling of his story? There was the somewhat cynical suggestion that 'blackboard' and 'black coffee' were not PC. Cynical yes, but seriously considered and even acted upon by some. Then there are the hitherto law-abiding citizens who find themselves in trouble with the police while the criminals they confronted are treated as the innocent party.

In fact, the politically correct pendulum has swung so much in favour of anyone not in the majority that it gives rise to totally irrational decision-making. When a hairdresser advertised for a 'Junior Stylist' she was told she was being unfair to anyone not considered 'junior'. When a recruitment agency boss suggested an applicant for an NHS cleaning job should be 'reliable' she was accused of discriminating against those who were 'unreliable'.

The people we rely on to be there when we need them have not escaped. Police officers are told how to ride their bikes safely and how to climb stepladders. Emergency services can't rush to our aid immediately because they have orders to find out just how much of an emergency it is, assess the risks to them and fill out forms first.

And where would this Fool Britannia state be without its endless list of obscure job titles with litter wardens being called Area Environmental Inspectors and the BBC, once the 'Bible' of our language, now creating jobs such as Solutions Architect and Organisational Development and Change Director. To be fair, it is not just the good old Beeb who has created a whole new language. There are the official gobbledy-gookers too, who would rather use the phrases 'blue sky thinking', 'bottom up' and 'funding streams' when 'new ideas', 'listening to people' and 'money' not only suffice, but are actually understood.

Much used, greatly abused. But what is the 'official' definition of Political Correctness? Here we go:

'Political correctness (adjectivally, politically correct; both forms commonly abbreviated to PC) is a term denoting language, ideas, policies, and behaviour seen as seeking to minimize social and institutional offence in occupational, gender, racial, cultural, sexual orientation, handicap, and age-related contexts. In current usage, the terms are almost exclusively pejorative, connoting "intolerant" and "intolerance" whilst the usage politically incorrect, denotes an implicitly positive self-description. Examples include the conservative *Politically Incorrect Guides* published by the Regnery editorial house and the television talk show *Politically Incorrect*. Thus, "politically incorrect" connotes language, ideas, and behaviour, unconstrained by orthodoxy and the fear of giving offence.'

The short dictionary definition is:
1. Of, relating to, or supporting broad social, political, and educational change, especially to redress historical injustices in matters such as race, class, gender, and sexual orientation.
2. Being or perceived as being over concerned with such change, often to the exclusion of other matters.

It was the 'New Left' who adopted the term 'political correctness' around 1970, later adapting its use to refer to satirical self-criticism. (In the early 1980s, feminists used it as a sarcastic reference to the anti-pornography movement's efforts to define 'feminist sexuality'.) Widespread use of the phrase 'politically

correct' came about in the 1990s when it was used as a derogatory term by the political right. Writing in the *New York Times* in
1990, Richard Bernstein said the term 'with its Stalinist orthodoxy is spoken more with irony and disapproval than with
reverence. But across the country the term PC as it is commonly
abbreviated, is being heard more and more in debates over what
should be taught in universities.'

As we know, it was downhill from then, with 'firemen'
becoming 'firefighters' and a chairman becoming a chairperson
(so as to become 'gender neutral') and blind and disabled people
being called 'visually challenged' and 'physically challenged'.
The word 'Christmas' has been deemed non-PC in some circumstances, replaced on batches of cards and posters with the word
'Holiday' inserted so as not to offend those who do not celebrate
this great, traditional and much-loved time of year.

Even traditional nursery rhymes like *Baa Baa Black Sheep*
– written in 1744 satirising the taxes imposed on wool exports –
has fallen foul of political correctness. In 2000 Birmingham City
Council tried to ban the rhyme, after claiming that it was racist
and portrayed negative stereotypes. The council rescinded the
ban after black parents said it was ludicrous. Margaret
Morrissey, of the National Confederation of Parent Teacher
Associations, said at the time: 'It's really sad. Children for generations have loved and enjoyed nursery rhymes and it's very sad
if adult political correctness doesn't allow them to grow up in an
unbiased world.'

This did not stop nursery schools in Oxfordshire several years
later altering *Baa Baa Black Sheep* to read *Baa Baa Rainbow Sheep*.
They also liked the way the children could 'turn the song into an
action rhyme . . . They sing happy, sad, bouncing, hopping, pink,
blue, black and white sheep etc.' The decision to change such a
traditional children's rhyme was, *The Times* reported: 'made
after the nurseries decided to re-evaluate their approach to equal
opportunities.' Stuart Chamberlain, manager of the Family

Centre in Abingdon and the Sure Start centre in Sutton Courtenay, Oxfordshire, told the local *Courier Journal* newspaper: 'We have taken the equal opportunities approach to everything we do. This is fairly standard across nurseries. We are following stringent equal opportunities rules. No one should feel pointed out because of their race, gender or anything else.' In keeping with the new approach, teachers at the nurseries changed the ending of *Humpty Dumpty* so as not to upset the children by Humpty's shell-shocked demise, and dropped the seven dwarfs from the title of *Snow White* because 'dwarf' was derogatory to height-challenged people. A spokesman for schools' watchdog Ofsted confirmed that centres are expected to 'have regard to anti-discrimination good practice' and that staff should 'actively promote equality of opportunity'.

As one commentator noted in 2007: 'Critics of PC have been accused of displaying the same sensitivity to word choice that they claim to oppose, and of perceiving non-existent political agenda.'

In 2009 we had the Equality Bill which reinforced the need not to discriminate. Commenting on the Bill, social observer and journalist Polly Toynbee said: 'The phrase "political correctness" was born as a coded cover for all who still want to say Paki, spastic or queer, all those who still want to pick on anyone not like them, playground bullies who never grew up. The politically correct society is the civilised society, however much some may squirm at the more inelegant official circumlocutions designed to avoid offence.' She added that the phrase 'is an empty right-wing smear designed only to elevate its user'. (The year 2009 was also, incidentally, the start of Britain's Great Wheelie Bin Revolt when householders rebelled against local councils' determination to control and monitor what we put in our refuse bins. Yes, Big Brother, with its sinister bureaucratic aim of keeping tabs on our very ordinary habits has also grabbed us firmly in its hand with wheelie bin inspectors, almost nationwide blanket CCTV surveillance and our details indiscriminately kept on databases.)

You will see in this book that victims of over-zealous political correctness often use the phrase 'political correctness gone mad'. They are quite right of course. You might take comfort in the fact that other countries have the term 'politically correct' too – and impress your friends by saying that in Scandinavia it is 'politiskt korrekt', in Italy 'politicamente corretto' and in Poland 'poprawny politycznie'.

Great Britain? More like Grate-on-your-nerves Britain. Feel free to peruse this book and see just how ludicrous our world of political correctness has become. There's no law against browsing – well not yet, anyway.

1

Aisle Be Blowed

When Krys Gunton decided to pop into her local Tesco store after a morning's riding, the one thing she did not expect was to be saddled with the insult of being called 'smelly'. Neither did she expect to be asked to leave the shop, Tesco Metro in Romford, Essex.

Miss Gunton had walked into the shop wearing jodhpurs and boots, having just finished an enjoyable hour on her horse Monty. But she was confronted by a security guard who asked her to leave on the grounds of health and safety because she apparently 'smelled too much'. Said Miss Gunton: 'At first I didn't understand him. But then it became clear that someone else in the shop complained about the smell to him. He kept repeating "You're smelling too much." I asked him what he thought I should do about it and he suggested I should change my clothes. I just told him that I didn't have any spare clothes and that there was nowhere to change anyway. The whole situation was completely ridiculous.'

A spokesman for Tesco said of the incident in January 2009: 'We apologise for any confusion or upset caused but we did ask the customer to leave for health and safety reasons. The customer was asked politely to leave the store as she had manure on her riding boots which is of course not acceptable in a store which sells food.' Miss Gunton, a 29-year-old university administrator, was adamant that there was no horse muck on her – only mud – and added: 'Before I went in I made sure I wasn't trailing mess everywhere. It was not like I was covered in horse muck. It was just "eau de horse!" I was totally humiliated in front of a shop full of people and felt forced to dump my shopping and simply walk out of there.'

Tesco hit the news again that month when 49-year-old Maurice Harris was forced to prove he was over 18 before the shop in Bedworth, Warwickshire would sell him a bag of party poppers. And in Tesco's in Chelmsford, a 23-year-old policeman was refused a bottle of wine because his partner with him was only 18. At yet another Tesco store, this time in Flitwick, Bedfordshire, a 48-year-old woman was asked to prove she was over 18 before she could buy a T-shirt bearing a Guinness logo. Oh, and good old Tesco hit the headlines in February when a 9-year-old girl with learning difficulties was banned from carrying a helium balloon into its superstore on the Tower Park leisure complex in Poole, Dorset. Little Alex Pearson had been given the balloon after enjoying a meal at the nearby Chiquito Mexican restaurant. Her mum, 44-year-old Marion Pearson, tied the balloon to Alex's wrist so it would not blow away before they entered the Tesco shop. But they were stopped by a security guard who said it was a health and safety risk. Said Mrs Pearson: 'Alex didn't understand why she wasn't allowed in and I told the security guard to explain it to her. He couldn't even look her in the eye. I think he was too embarrassed.' A Tesco spokesman said that on that day a number of children had come into the store and let the balloons loose either accidentally or deliberately. 'Unfortunately they were getting trapped on the ceiling and blocking the sprinkler system and they are pretty difficult to retrieve. The managers decided to use their discretion.' In November a group of students, all over 18, went to the Tesco store in Warwick to buy a bottle of wine, a birthday cake and a packet of candles. They were asked for ID, which six could produce but one couldn't. So the cashier refused to sell them the wine. They said they would just take the cake and the candles then. Sorry, said the cashier, but you can't have the candles, either. Why not? No ID. The students were left with just the cake.

Standing 6 feet tall and aged 20, Stephen Stuart never experienced any problems over looking his age – except when he tried to buy a 12A-rated DVD from his local Sainsbury store in Didcot, Oxfordshire, in October. Despite sporting stubble and looking anything but a lad less than 12 years old, Stephen was nevertheless refused his purchase of the *X-Men Origins: Wolverine* DVD when he could not produce any ID. Said Stephen: 'I asked the girl at the till: "Do I look 11 or under?" The last thing I thought I would need to buy a 12A DVD at my age and height was ID. If I was buying a bottle of whisky or an X-rated film I'd understand. But this was a DVD about a comic superhero. I get served in pubs and clubs without a glance . . .' After the cashier and a supervisor both refused to sell Stephen the £9.99 DVD, his 53-year-old dad Ian took over the transaction – after cheekily showing his driving licence. 'She told me not to be so silly,' said Ian. A spokesman for Sainsbury's commented: 'Customers who look under 25 are asked for ID on age-related items and that includes all DVDs.' A similar incident happened at the Marks & Spencer store in South Mimms when Andree Evans bought a birthday card and the till automatically sounded the 'check they are over 25' alarm because the card had a picture of bottles of wine, wine glasses and a corkscrew.

Still in the silly department of over-the-counter craziness, 15-year-old Jaz Bhogal was banned from buying a bag of wine gums at a discount store in Wisbech, Cambridgeshire because he needed to be 18-plus to buy anything containing alcohol. Jaz was even chased down the street with his purchase, ordered to return to the 99p Store and had his sweets confiscated. He was, however, refunded his 99p. Said Jaz: 'I couldn't believe it. I was asked how old I was and when I said I was 15, I was told they couldn't sell me the sweets. They said they had wine in them and pointed to the word "wine" on the packet. I was absolutely speechless.' Added mum Sue, 36: 'I thought Jaz was joking when he came home and told me what had happened. It is ridiculous and I would have been really cross if I had asked him to buy them for me.' Wine gums, of course, do not contain wine. A spokesman for 99p Stores admitted: 'Because the Wisbech store opened fairly recently there seems to have been an unfortunate glitch. We have rectified this and are sure it will not happen again at any of our UK stores.' He added: 'To show that we have a good sense of humour we would like to offer Jaz a nine-item voucher in the store – on condition that at least one of those products is wine gums . . .'

When 70-year-old retired oil worker Chris Pether tried to buy two lemons at the self-service checkout at the Asda store in Aberdeen, he was greeted with a message telling him he had bought too many. Obviously a little taken aback by this, Mr Pether sought the assistance of a shop supervisor who told him that because teenagers tended to throw fruit at people, health and safety rules now prevented them from selling more than one loose lemon, orange or grapefruit. Even more bizarre, the pensioner was told he could buy a bag of ten lemons because they weren't 'loose' and were smaller, meaning their potential as a lethal weapon was lessened. He didn't take up the offer, instead choosing to turn his lemon purchase into two separate transactions and thereby getting round the rules. Said Mr Pether: 'It takes some believing. It was so ludicrous but it's part and parcel of the expansion of the nanny state.' Commented a spokesman for Asda: 'It sounds like one of our colleagues was having a really bad day. People can buy as many lemons, oranges and grapefruits as they like.'

Despite her protests, management consultant Jackie Slater was not allowed to purchase two bottles of wine because she was in the company of her 17-year-old daughter and 18-year-old niece – who the staff at the Morrison's store in Leeds thought Mrs Slater might be buying the alcohol for. She was asked to show some ID and was quizzed by an assistant about the two young girls chatting at the end of the checkout. Said Mrs Slater: 'I told her I was really flattered, but I was the wrong side of 50 . . . the assistant asked "Are they with you?" I said they'd come to help me carry the bags back to the car. The assistant said: "You could be buying the wine for them. It's the policy – I have to see everyone's ID to make sure they are all over 18." I was embarrassed, there was a huge queue building up and my daughter found it all excruciating,' said Mrs Slater, who describes the incident as 'the silliest bit of jobsworth nonsense' she had ever come across. 'It comes to something when a mother can't take her daughter shopping without being made to feel like a criminal.' In vain, Mrs Slater insisted that the wine was for herself and her husband, Peter. But the assistant and then the store manager refused to budge. Morrison's head office backed the store with a spokesman saying: 'Under current licensing laws, stores are unable to sell an alcoholic product to a customer they believe could be buying for a minor or for someone who is unable to prove their age. We take our responsibility with regard to selling alcohol very seriously. The rules are in place to protect our customers and their families, as well as local communities who, in the majority of cases, appreciate our vigilance in the sale of age-restricted products.' But the company did not contest Mrs Slater's version of events. The assistant even agreed that she would have sold the wine to a mother who had younger children with her because 'no one would buy wine for a 12-year-old'.

A misunderstanding over a mum's support of British troops injured while fighting in Afghanistan led to her being refused service at an Asda store in Rochdale. Beth Hoyle was wearing a Help for Heroes wristband which was sadly interpreted by an Asian cashier as the mother of three supporting war in both Afghanistan and Iraq. He was backed up by a store supervisor who told Beth the cashier was entitled to his point of view and to refuse to serve her 'because of what she was wearing'. Said Beth: 'I told him it was nothing to do with the war, but about supporting injured troops. I complained to a supervisor, but he said it was his right not to serve me. I was disgusted.' A spokesman for Asda said they were 'shocked' by the claim but could not find any evidence of the incident taking place, adding that the supermarket chain was a supporter of Help for Heroes and sold its campaign wristbands and badges.

In a separate incident, staff at the Asda store on Hayling Island, Hampshire, asked 61-year-old Ed Spencer to verify he was over 18 before he was allowed to buy a can of non-alcoholic shandy.

It seemed the obvious thing to do . . . Sue Savage, a little on the short side and in an ankle brace after breaking her leg, asked her much taller daughter Tara to stretch up to pick vodka and rum mixers from a high shelf at their local Co-op store in Cranbrook, Kent. But when she tried to pay, Mrs Savage was accused of trying to supply alcohol to a minor. Already a bit stressed over the cocktail party she was planning, she tried to explain why she was buying the drink. But a supervisor insisted she leave the bottles of booze in the shop. The mother-of-two later returned on her own to have another go but was told again – this time by the shop manager – that it was believed she was buying drink for a minor. Thoroughly frustrated now, Mrs Savage threw a £10 note on the counter and left with her purchases, with the warning she was breaking the law ringing in her ears. Now in a complete dither, she called the police for advice. They arrived two hours later, advised her to return the drink, arrested her and gave her an £80 fixed penalty notice. Determined to take the matter further, she stormed: 'It's ridiculous. Does this mean anyone with children cannot go shopping with them and buy alcohol?' A spokesman for the Co-op said: 'We are a respectable retailer and have a legal responsibility to ensure that alcohol is not sold to children.'

Queries over customers' age when buying an item with even a slight relation to alcohol or when some other loony PC bit of legislation comes into play is commonplace nowadays. But even then, it was hard to work out why 24-year-old office worker Christine Cuddihy had a Tesco checkout cashier quibbling over a 51p slice of quiche – because Christine 'looked under 21'. The bizarre shopping experience happened at the Tesco store in Cannons Park, Coventry, in January 2010 when Christine, from nearby Leamington Spa, popped in to buy the quiche for her supper. Tesco, as we already know, have a rather strange approach to customer relations sometimes. On this occasion the cashier told Christine that she could not go through the checkout with her quiche because of the doubts about her age, saying: 'You don't look over 21. I need some proof of age.' Christine obviously queried this and was met with the response: 'We have to be really strict now and this applies to quiche bought over the counter.' There was something of a heated debate between the two women, but eager to avoid further embarrassment with a queue growing longer behind her, Christine produced her driving licence and fled. She naturally had much to say about the surreal encounter. 'It was very embarrassing. What on earth is dangerous about a slice of quiche? There was nothing suspicious about me and it's not even like I was buying a whole quiche to binge on. It was rush-hour and the shop was really busy. I was so insulted that they thought I couldn't be trusted with a harmless snack. I was really embarrassed and just wanted to get out of the shop. The irony of the whole thing is that I've bought alcohol from there dozens of times without being asked for ID. I've racked my brains to come up with an explanation but I can't find one. The whole thing is ridiculous.' Tesco later apologised and admitted shoppers did not have to prove their age when they bought quiche. Confessed a spokesman: 'We're at a loss to say what happened here. We couldn't find the staff member who asked for the ID. Age-related prompts at till are set centrally and there obviously isn't one on quiche.'

. . . But is there a Tesco policy of treating all teenagers as prospective thieves? The question had to be asked when in February it was revealed that staff at the Tesco Express store in Halesowen in the West Midlands were ordering school-children to remove their blazers and deposit their bags at a checkpoint before they were allowed in to buy snacks. One witness was horrified, saying: 'I feel it is inappropriate for an adult to ask teenage boys and girls to remove clothing and trust them with their possessions, especially as all teenagers and schoolchildren were being branded thieves. When confronted, a senior member of staff at the store replied: "Don't tell me. I'm just the manager." ' One feels the schoolchildren could have got their own back by pointing out the spelling mistakes in a sign warning about the new policy: 'Due to issues anybody in school uniform will be asked to leave there jacket/blazer and bags by the front door unless accomipant with an adult.' Defending the policy a Tesco spokesman said: 'We take our responsibilities seriously. We've had a number of issues in this store and complaints from other customers. We have discussed this with the local school and have regretfully had to restrict the number of schoolchildren coming into the store.' Founder of the lobby group Parents Outloud, Margaret Morrisey, did not accept this explanation, saying: 'It is a horrible policy, effectively saying that all the children are thieves. It would be far better to have staff keep a close eye on them, or limit the number of pupils allowed in at once. If there is a problem, surely it would have been better for the managers to talk to the school and have it dealt with. You can't get young people to take clothes off to enter a shop. It is just not right.'

2

No More Fun and Games

The Performing Rights Society, a group which fiercely protects the performance of artistes' music unless a fee is paid, came down heavily on car mechanic Len Attwood in January. Was he singing to an audience? Was he playing music at a gathering? No. Len was simply beavering away in his workshop when raided by the PRS. He was accused of not displaying one of their stickers to prove he had a licence to play their music on a radio in public. Except Len did not have a radio. The PRS hit back with the retort that even if Len did not have a radio, his customers would have them in their cars, and of course, they may not always turn them off upon arrival. Len was ordered to buy a licence or put up a prominent notice ordering motorists to switch off all in-car entertainment before driving through the door. A similar incident happened when Sandra Burt was singing quite happily as she worked behind the counter at the A & T village shop in Clackmannanshire, Scotland. One of the reasons Mrs Burt wanted to sing was because the shop had already been contacted some months before to warn them that a licence was needed if they had a radio playing for customers. It was an expense the shop could not afford so the radio had to go. A visit from the music police over Mrs Burt's singing ended with the demand for £80 for a performing rights licence. Said a very determined Gareth Kelly, music sales advisor for PRS: 'Using any copyright material in your store, without paying for it, is illegal. It doesn't matter whether you're singing a Robbie Williams track, or listening to a Robbie Williams track, you still have to pay for it.' He added that Mrs Burt could be fined 'for not having a live performance licence, and if the fine isn't paid, then she could potentially be taken to court'. He also added that under the PRS rules, 56-year-old Mrs Burt could be judged to be giving daily performances, which would require individual daily licences, taking the annual cost up to 'four figures'. Said Mrs Burt: 'I would start to sing to myself when I was stacking the shelves just to keep me happy because it was very quiet without the radio. When I heard that the PRS said I would be prosecuted for not having a performance licence, I thought it was a joke and started laughing. I was then told I could be fined thousands of pounds. But I couldn't stop myself singing. They would need to put a plaster over my mouth to get me to stop, I can't help it.' A later apology from the PRS after the story hit the headlines was music to Mrs Burt's ears. She was sent a bouquet of flowers and a note that said: 'We're very sorry we made a big mistake. We hear you have a lovely singing voice and we wish you good luck.'

For football fans, it's all part of the fun – cheering your team on from the stands and generally making your presence known. But supporters of Premier League club Middlesbrough were silenced in their seats after the club decreed fans could only cheer if the team scored – a rare event considering there was one time when it failed to find the net for eight hours and plunged into the relegation zone.

The 'hush' orders came from Middlesbrough's safety officer Sue Watson who also asked fans not to stand up too much during games. In her note, Ms Watson wrote: 'I am receiving more and more complaints from our own fans about both the persistent standing and the constant banging and noise coming from the back of the stand. Please stop. Make as much noise as you like when we score, but this constant noise is driving some fans mad.'

Stunned supporters couldn't believe it when they read the new club rules before a match at the club's Riverside Stadium in

February (which incidentally ended in a 0–0 draw, so no cheers there). Said one fan: 'It's a passionate sport. Are they going to give us prompt cards to tell us when we can sing and when we can't? You'd think that given our current league position the club would be wanting us to help rally the team.'

Following a furore about the silent orders on Facebook, the club's chief operating officer Neil Bausor backed down, saying: 'We understand the strength of feeling on this issue and accept the letter could easily have been misunderstood. We apologise to any supporters who have therefore been understandably annoyed.'

They have graced floats, processions and the opening of local events for many years. Little girls aspire to be one. And parents are quite rightly proud to see their daughter crowned as one. But as far as Weymouth in Dorset is concerned, Carnival Queens are sexist and should no longer be allowed. Instead of retaining a pretty girl with a lovely smile and waving hand, a politically-correct group has decided there should be a Carnival Community Champion, a male or female 'unsung hero'. The decision was made in March 2009 by the Weymouth Community Volunteers who took over running the local carnival from the Round Table. New carnival organiser Sue Follan said: 'The carnival queen contest is a closed shop as it only applies to glamorous young women and we think it is time for a change . . .'

It's been a great British tradition, perhaps viewed by some as not the greatest of pursuits, but train-spotting has always been with us – until security fears went off the rails in March 2009. Retired accountant Edmund Tan, 54, was told to stop taking photographs at Macclesfield station by Virgin Rail staff who said he was a 'security risk'. The company said it feared possible terrorist attacks.

But said a perplexed Mr Tan who came to Britain from Hong Kong in 1972: 'I have never encountered anything like this apart from once in China, which is a communist country. Is Britain really becoming a country like that? It is really very frightening.'

The ban was instigated by National Express and includes London's King's Cross station, Stevenage, Peterborough, Doncaster, Leeds, Wakefield, Newcastle upon Tyne and Durham stations. Concerned over the stringent rules, Gerry Doherty, general secretary of rail union TSSA said: 'Do they really think that a 10-year-old boy with a pencil and notebook is in possession of a dangerous weapon? You do wonder what planet these people are on. Young train-spotters have been with us since Victorian times. Now National Express is saying they should be banned because they are a nuisance.'

Film footage of Mr Tan showed him pleading with the Virgin staff member who he said was 'very rude' and who in turn accused him of 'being abusive'.

But Virgin Trains were unrepentant. A spokesman said that Mr Tan could not take photographs without permission – and that permission was not going to be given, adding: 'There are a number of issues around security. They could include things like terrorism or security of the station.'

It was all sad news for Mr Tan who says he loves trains and has over 200 model trains at his home in Prestbury, Cheshire.

A wave of political correctness gone mad hit London Fields Lido in Hackney, East London, in March when swimmers were told it was too wet to take the plunge.

They were informed that they would be banned if it started to rain. And that is just what happened when there was a downpour and they were told to wait outside until it was over.

Said one baffled swimmer: 'It was difficult to believe that what I was hearing was serious. The idea that it could be too wet to swim seems almost incredible but that was what they were actually saying.' Hackney Council justified its decision by saying: 'In exceptional circumstances the pool may be required to be closed in order to protect users' safety. For example, exceptionally heavy rain or foggy conditions can distort the clarity of the water, restricting lifeguards' visibility and their ability to keep swimmers safe.'

Stunned objectors felt the tide of health and safety rules was turning – and not for the good. Said Conservative MP Patrick Mercer: 'This rule is ridiculous and the ultimate example of risk avoidance. If we continue down this mad path of mindless health and safety rules it will get even worse. There's no common sense and this is just a continuation of the growing nanny state that prevents people doing more and more things.'

Around the same time, managers at Crystal Palace National Sports Centre in south London barred the public from swimming in half of the pool's eight lanes because of fears lifeguards may not be able to see them properly. This was despite staff insisting that they had never experienced that problem.

The opening of the prestigious cricket event, the Ashes test, in July presented a sticky wicket for political correctness. It was decreed that three anthems and two hymns would be sung so as not to offend any participants. That meant that the England team facing Australia in Cardiff, Wales, would stand to the Welsh national anthem as well as singing God Save The Queen. A singer was brought in to perform the Australian national anthem, Advance Australia Fair. Just for good measure, soprano Katherine Jenkins was called upon by Glamorgan County Cricket Club to sing the Welsh hymn Calon Lan – as well as the Welsh national anthem. Yet another singer was summoned to sing Jerusalem, a firm favourite among England supporters. One assumes that the match eventually got under way. Proclaimed former umpire Dickie Bird: 'This is absolutely ridiculous and didn't happen in my day. They should just stick to one anthem if they feel they have to have them. Otherwise it becomes a bit of a farce and they'll be lucky to get play under way before lunch starts.'

It has long been one of the delights of parenting – watching your children having fun in the local playground. But the innocent and perfectly natural activity was blighted in October when parents were banned from supervising their children at play in two playgrounds in Watford, Hertfordshire, in case they were paedophiles. A notice from Watford Borough Council claimed that because of Ofsted regulations, every authorised adult who enters the grounds must now be vetted and undergo a Criminal Records Bureau check. Said Watford Mayor, Dorothy Thornhill: 'Sadly, in today's climate, you can't have adults wandering around unchecked in a children's playground. We have reviewed our procedures, so although previously some parents have stayed with their children at the discretion of play workers, this is not something we can continue to do.' Instead, rangers 'patrolled' the two parks where the skateboarding, zip-wires, rope swings and other activities are aimed at 5 to 15-year-olds. Stormed one mother: 'I find it insulting that the council are branding everyone paedophiles and telling us we cannot be trusted with our own kids. It's a disgrace. They have some pen-pusher sitting behind a desk telling good people they can't spend quality time with their children.' Ofsted said the guidelines had been misunderstood and agreed that the presence of parents 'can be an important part of children settling in somewhere new'. Added a spokesman for children's charity Kidscape: 'Caring parents should not be viewed as a threat. A parent or carer is in a better position to look after their children than council staff.'

You would have thought that if Disney's classic film *101 Dalmatians* was going to be the focus of any ban, it would be because of the terrifying threat of puppies being turned into fur coats. But in August, when the film was at the centre of controversy, it had nothing to do with animal rights protestors (though we guess had they thought about it, they would have got in first) but anti-smokers. It was decreed that an 18 certificate – usually reserved for films with violent and sexual content – would be slapped on any film featuring smoking. And, as any *101 Dalmatians* fan will know, the wicked fur-loving Cruella de Vil was never without a cigarette in its long holder. The ban will mainly target new releases but will affect older animated films such as *Dalmatians*, *Peter Pan* and *The Little Mermaid*, if they are reissued and reclassified – meaning the children's films can only be seen by 'children' over 18 . . . Classics such as *Casablanca*, *Titanic* and *Lord of the Rings* would also have the restricted viewing, brought in by Liverpool City Council, which declared it would only give a lower age rating to films which gave 'a clear and unambiguous portrayal of the dangers of smoking, other tobacco use, or second-hand smoke'. The British Board of Film Classification is generally responsible for classifying films but under the Licensing Act 2003, local councils have the powers to decide on the rating of films shown in their area. Commented Tory local Government spokesman, Bob Neill: 'This is a sledge-hammer to crack a nut. It is not the role of town halls to act as puritanical thought police, banning children from watching films like *Lord of the Rings*, *101 Dalmatians* and *Casablanca* because they offend politically correct sensibilities.'

It took four years to recreate a wood and paper flying machine that once soared in the air 100 years ago. It took just a moment for killjoys to put an end to any idea of the £10,000 modern-day machine taking to the skies. For although back in 1909 a triplane built by Alliott Verdon-Roe safely flew 100 feet at an altitude of 20 feet, propelled by a nine-horse engine, such a craft was deemed as not airworthy in today's times. The creative team of retired engineers and members of the Manchester Museum of Science and Industry were told that to make their plane safe, they had to use a man-made material called seconite instead of paper, install a harness for the pilot and make adjustments to the propeller. All of which made the plane somewhat heavier than the original – and therefore unable to fly anyway. Said disappointed project leader Mike Taylor: 'I don't think we had enough power out of the engine. The original was fragile and every time Alliott Verdon-Roe had it out he broke something. He didn't have health and safety rules to meet. As soon as our replica gets in the air the law says it must be airworthy.'

                                        *   *   *

Oh, the warmth and the roar of a bonfire on Guy Fawkes Night!
Throw another piece of wood on . . . well, that's what we've all
been doing for centuries, much to the delight of young and old
alike. And even if public fires and firework displays have been
actively encouraged over the years rather than private back
garden ones (health and safety of course!) then it has all still
been good fun. Except at Ilfracombe Rugby Club, Devon, in
November 2009. It was not so much light the blue touch-paper
and withdraw but more a case of pushing a button. For the
club's bonfire was shown in all its glory on a giant television
screen after it got fed up with battling all the health and safety
rules over having a real fire. North Devon Council had
demanded that the night's traditional entertainment could only
take place if there were five qualified marshals on duty and
metal barriers in place. It was acting after an incident some years
earlier when yobs threw fireworks at another sports club
bonfire. Hence, what was described as 'non-bonfire night' by
some disgruntled spectators involved a 16ft by 12ft £2,500
screen showing a roaring bonfire – complete with giant heaters,
lighting, sounds of crackling wood and a smoke machine. Said
the rugby club's captain, Lee Cooper, 25: 'Certain regulations
make it difficult for us to have a real bonfire . . . so we tried to
come up with an original, imaginative and fun way to fill the
void. The bonfire is often the focal point so we decided to have
a big screen that would do the same job.' Attending families
were allowed to wave sparklers at the screen. Nothing about the
'virtual bonfire' was quite the same as the real thing and as one
visitor said: 'The whole point of Guy Fawkes Night is to watch
and smell a real bonfire. I doubt Guy Fawkes would have been
able to blow up Parliament with virtual gunpowder . . .'

There have not been too many reports of serious mishaps while
feeding ducks (indeed, have there been any at all?) but that did
not stop Sandwell Council in the West Midlands from ruining
the day for Vanessa Kelly and her 17-month-old boy Harry. Her

trip to Smethwick Hall Park ended with her being served an on-the-spot £75 fine for spreading litter (bread) and with a female park warden requesting the young mother stop feeding the ducks immediately because there had been complaints about children slipping on duck mess. But while 26-year-old Ms Kelly – who pointed out there were no health and safety signs up to warn would-be duck feeders – was ordered to stop handing bread to the ducks, her toddler was allowed to carry on as he was too young to prosecute. Said Ms Kelly: 'I take my son to feed the ducks every week. He loves it. It is just for his entertainment and to keep him happy. It is doing a good deed as the ducks are obviously looking for the food.' She announced she was refusing to pay the fine, took photographs to show the absence of warning signs and lodged a complaint with Sandwell Council. Councillor Mahboob Hussain, the council cabinet member for neighbourhoods and housing, strongly supported the local council's stance in a long, long statement, saying: 'We have had so many complaints about problems caused by the feeding of pigeons and waterfowl that we decided to create designated feeding areas for birds. We have done a lot of educational work to get this message across and we have warned people not to feed them other than in the designated areas. This park has a problem with Canada Geese and people living nearby have made many complaints about them. They feel intimidated by the large numbers of geese. Many road-users also feel the birds are a danger to motorists as they regularly obstruct the road. We are taking this very seriously and acting on these complaints. Too much food can cause bird populations to grow out of control as well as leaving litter and attracting rats which poses an environmental health risk.' A council spokesman added: 'As the woman was being issued with the fine, the kid was still throwing bread. In a temper she turned round and said "I suppose you're going to issue him with a fine as well".' Ms Kelly decided to take Harry to a park where feeding ducks would not lead to her getting a big 'bill' . . .

* * *

Bingo! The political correctness that has now encompassed Britain hit one of the nation's best-loved pastimes in December 2009. Sudbury Town Council in Suffolk banned the traditional bingo-caller's phrases of 'two fat ladies' for the number 88 and 'legs eleven' for the number 11 with the view that it could be sued by overweight players or women who claimed sexism. That meant that when he hosted the traditional Tuesday afternoon session in the town hall 75-year-old John Sayers had to stick to a 'numbers only' ruling. As political correctness critic, Richard Littlejohn, asked: 'Does this mean that we can no longer say "Kelly's Eye" for the number one in case we offend the visually challenged?' The ruling saw the regular turnout of around 100 players drop, meaning so too, did the money they raised for charity each year – around £3,000. The bingo-lovers instead went to play at the local village of Great Cornard where no-one objected to 'two fat ladies' or anything else for that matter. Said Mr Sayers, a Sudbury town, district and county councillor: 'I was disappointed but I took good advice. I did not want to bring the town hall and myself into disrespect.' But a spokesman for the Plain English Campaign commented: 'Although banning bingo terms may sound quite humorous at first, it does have very serious implications. Political correctness was something that was brought in to establish fairness and equality, but it has in fact taken things to the other extreme.'

Father Christmas is one who knows that reindeer are more than sure-footed in the snow. After all, they manage to get around the Arctic Circle without too much trouble. Unfortunately, the quaint Leicestershire town of Market Harborough was deemed too dangerous for Rudolph and his eight pals in the case of snowfall – and the antlered guests were cancelled. It was just three hours before the reindeer were due to arrive at the town square that posters were put up ending the event with the words: 'There is a risk of slips and falls to attendees at the event, when the conditions get worse.' It was believed that cancelling the reindeers' appearance cost the taxpayer around £10,000.

Stormed Malcolm Lever-Jones, Independent Traders Association spokesman: 'It is health and safety gone barmy and completely ruined the festive mood. Hundreds of people had come from up to 40 miles away and were dreadfully disappointed. The council said there was a risk of snow and ice to pedestrians but with or without the reindeer, the streets were still icy. None of the town centre was cordoned off. It just made no sense.' Justifying their actions, a spokesman for Harborough Council said: 'Obviously, the reindeer would have loved the snow. But sadly we decided to cancel because of the possible danger to people, including young children.'

It was good enough for Forties music hall star George Formby (for those of us old enough to remember!) but it was not good enough for the Ofsted inspectors who visited New Road primary school in Sowerby Bridge, West Yorkshire in January 2010. They decreed that the ukulele was not a proper musical instrument – despite the school band being so good it was invited to play at Blackpool's famous Tower Ballroom. The inspectors said that the children's ukulele lessons – provided by an outside service – did not represent a wide enough musical experience for the youngsters even though the children themselves said they loved them. The official report stated: 'Music lessons and the curriculum do not provide sufficient challenge and, as a result, pupils do not make adequate progress. Achievement in music is inadequate.' Said one unhappy parent: 'The band is good and it sounds wonderful no matter what Ofsted says. The children were very upset at the criticism and they are all learning to read music as a result which is just wonderful. Who do these people think they are coming into good schools and making everyone feel awful?' Head teacher Charles Rowland defended the lessons too, adding: 'We do well in terms of opportunities for music beyond the classroom and we have an action plan to improve classroom teaching which involves providing the service ourselves. By Easter, we expect to be delivering music lessons which are at least satisfactory to inspectors.'

*   *   *

In early February 2010, visitors to twelfth-century Delapre Abbey, Northamptonshire, were banned from drinking tea in the gardens – because they slurped too loudly. At a meeting of Northampton Borough Council's planning committee, it was decided the tea-drinking caused a disturbance in the quiet grounds and that the tables and chairs outside the tea room should be removed and relocated to an area formerly used as a car park. This was after planning officer Andrew Holden told the meeting: 'We want to keep the walled garden as a peaceful space and it was being disturbed by tea-drinking.' The Abbey, set in 600 acres of park and farmland attracts around 120,000 visitors a year – many of whom looked forward to a traditional pot of tea for two – £3.20 with a slice of cake. The decision did not please everyone. Mr Graham Walker, 61, and chairman of the Friends of Delapre Abbey said it was petty, adding: 'Because we are ruining the ambience, we are going to be stuck in the car park instead of our beautiful walled garden. We are a charity which has made a fantastic success of the abbey and we are being squeezed financially because the tea room is one of our biggest sources of revenue. The whole thing seems absolutely crazy and I hope we can work with the council to find a compromise.'

It all seems harmless enough – children having fun on St Valentine's Day. But teachers at Ashcombe Primary School in Weston-super-Mare, Somerset, decided pupils were too young to wear their heart on their sleeves – or indeed hide their 'crush' on another. The children were banned from sending cards on February 14th 2010. If any were found at school they would be confiscated. The order affected all the school's 430 pupils aged between 5 and 11. Explaining his actions, head teacher Peter Turner said: 'Some children and parents encourage a lot of talk about boyfriends and girlfriends. This often leads to children being upset when they are "dumped" and other fuss which interrupts their learning. The school believes that such ideas should wait until children are mature enough emotionally and socially to understand the commitment involved in having or being a boyfriend or girlfriend. For this reason, we do not wish to see any Valentine's Day cards in school this year . . .' Some parents did not agree, with one saying: 'Learning about relationships and forming bonds with others is an important part of school life. Children of all ages develop crushes and Valentine's Day is a harmless way for them to indulge those crushes in a fun manner . . .'

. . . Another age-old tradition was panned by St Albans City Council when it declared that pancake races were dangerous. Spectators at the Shrove Tuesday event in St Albans, Hertfordshire, booed tourism manager Charles Baker as he announced: 'We have a new set of rules today due to the wet weather conditions and health and safety regulations' – those regulations were that the pancake racers should now become pancake walkers to avoid falling over. Said one observer: 'When he made the announcement the crowd went crazy and booed. It wasn't even raining. It was just a bit wet on the ground. The rule made the whole thing quite dull because usually people belt up and down the course.' A member of one of the three teams who were disqualified for breaking the rules, commented: 'I have been disqualified from a running race for running.' The council stood its ground and said that the rules had been introduced because of rain and that the 'odd person' had slipped in the past – requiring a plaster. Said Laura Midgley of pressure group Campaign Against Political Correctness: 'There has got to be an acceptable level of risk. There is still a danger in walking, so should they start crawling to avoid tripping up?'

3

Oh Bother, It's Big Brother

The New Year started with a number of job vacancies – or jobsworth vacancies as some saw it. Topping the list of public sector 'non-jobs' was the £19,887 a year Street Football Co-ordinator post advertised by Moray Council in which the successful applicant would be in charge of showing children how to play football. Then came the Community Space Challenge Co-ordinator (£33,777 a year) for Southwark in south London who was needed to tell young people 'at risk of offending' how to use public spaces. Charnwood Borough Council's Head of Communities and Partnership was offered a salary of up to £37,543 a year to ensure that community issues are 'resolved with lasting solutions'. Anyone applying to Herts County Council's advert for Head of Participation and Inclusion (up to £42,197 a year) had the brief of encouraging people to play musical instruments. The £38,556 a year job of Climate Change Manager for Braintree Council was created to reduce the 'council's effect on the planet'. All of which prompted the TaxPayers' Alliance to retort: 'In times of economic hardship, it is vitally important that the public sector tightens its belt, just as families are having to. With the public finances in such a mess, tax-payers cannot afford for quangos and councils to splash out on "non-jobs" that would be an indulgence even in the economic good times.'

In January 2009, the 'food police' invaded the country with householders being quizzed on their doorsteps about the amount of food they threw away.

The idea was to reduce the amount of food which goes to waste each year – estimated at around £8billion. Officials paid by the Government-backed Waste and Resources Action Programme also offered hints on recipes using leftovers.

But critics of the £30,000 scheme thought it was, well, a waste . . . Said Mark Wallace, campaigns director of the TaxPayers' Alliance: 'This is a prime example of excessive Government nannying and a waste of public money and resources. We are in the middle of a recession where every penny is even more valuable. The last thing people need is someone bossing them about in their own kitchen. If the Government has money sloshing around it should give it back to the taxpayer.'

The 'food police' initially started with an eight-week trial in six areas with inspectors earning up to £8.49 an hour and visiting 24,500 homes. The scheme was set to be spread throughout the country later in the year.

Spy planes swooped over Norfolk in January to see if householders were wasting too much energy. The planes were equipped with thermal-imaging cameras which create colour-coded maps informing the council of wasteful offenders so that they can be advised to mend their ways.

Broadland District Council spent £30,000 on the scheme which critics said was a waste of money, time and energy in itself. Said Matthew Elliott, chief executive of the TaxPayers' Alliance: 'People are sick and tired of being spied on by local Government and this council has shown an utter disregard for the man on the street. We are in a recession and you would have thought this council would have better ways to spend £30,000.'

Broadland hired the plane for five days at the end of January. It took images of homes and businesses, with those losing the most heat showing up red and those that were better insulated appearing blue.

Defending the pilot scheme (which was said to be so successful other authorities wanted to follow) the council's head of environment services, Andy Jarvis, said: 'We realised it would be useful to see if any of the homes which were not particularly hot had not had loft insulation. We were also able to look at very cold properties and think we might have picked up people on low incomes who are not heating their homes because they cannot afford to.' Council leader Simon Woodbridge said the project would 'effectively pay for itself within a few weeks in terms of the amount of money we can help people to save'.

The first city in the UK to make a heat-loss map was Aberdeen, followed by London's Haringey Council in 2007.

Pensioner Hannah Humphris was bombarded with demands to buy a TV licence. They arrived regularly at her home in Neath, South Wales, culminating in the threat of prosecution and a possible fine of £1,000. You would have thought this would be enough to prompt the former shorthand typist into doing the right thing. Except she does not own a television – and indeed has not done so for nearly thirty years. And of course, Miss Humphris told TV Licensing this way back when her television broke down in 1978 and she never bought another. Despite her regular assurances that she did not have a TV, Miss Humphris was still sent a letter she described as 'intimidating' and 'threatening'. She even willingly agreed to a 'TV search' of her home by the authority. Said Miss Humphris: 'I think it must be amusing for them to keep harassing me like this. Am I a criminal now because I don't own a television set?' A spokesman for TV Licensing said Miss Humphris should not receive any more letters but that she may still receive a visit to check she is indeed without a television . . .

Stuart Kennedy is a stripagram, one of those people who turn up at a party, sing 'Happy Birthday' and then embarrass the 'victim' by taking their clothes off in front of them. Stuart's particular stripagram guise was as a policeman, 'Sergeant Eros', and he charged £115 a time in a bid to pay off his student loan . . . But the real policemen of Grampian did not like it. They

spent £170,000 over two years trying to convict Stuart for imper-
sonating a police officer. He had been arrested six times
between March 2007 and January 2009, and made twenty-two
court appearances – all ending without a single conviction. They
even tried to charge him with possessing an offensive weapon –
and that failed too.

Also early in 2009 Big Brother was keeping a beady eye on us all
buying the demon drink from shops and supermarkets. A law
was quietly pushed through Parliament giving councils the
power to order licensed premises – including pubs – to fit the
CCTV cameras. Police warned pubs that their licensing applications would not be supported unless they agreed to install the
cameras. The first blanket policy was introduced in the London
borough of Islington where all applicants wanting a licence to
sell alcohol were told they must fit CCTV. Other police forces are
taking the same stance.

   Footage of people buying alcohol must be stored for at least
sixty days and handed over to the police on demand. The whole
idea is to crack down on under-age drinking.

   But critics of the loss of personal freedom complained that the
good British public is now being tracked everywhere they go.
The UK already has more than 4 million surveillance cameras
covering the streets – the highest amount in the world.

   Some thought it was not quite right that Home Office Minister
Alan Campbell, who piloted the CCTV measures through the
House of Commons, confessed he could not remember the last
time he was in a pub . . .

   Mark Hastings, spokesman for the British Beer and Pub
Association stormed: 'It's an extraordinary admission from
someone who is proposing measures that, on the Government's
own admission, will cost the pub sector hundreds of thousands
of pounds a year. It shows how disconnected he is from the
realities of what it's like trying to stay in business in the current
environment.'

*   *   *

Who can ever forget those moments of passion in the classic film *Brief Encounter*? Well, jobsworth rail bosses at Warrington Bank Quay Station in Cheshire certainly have. They killed off romance in February by erecting 'no kissing' signs by the taxi rank to stop couples from holding up the queue. Passengers were told they could only shake hands while waiting in the taxi line. If they wanted to do more, they had to move on to a 'properly designated area'. The idea was that of Colin Daniels, chief executive of Warrington Chamber of Commerce who explained: 'It was all a bit of fun. But now Virgin Trains have agreed to put the signs up as part of a refurbishment. They may seem frivolous, but there is a serious message underneath. They certainly make our station unique.' The signs, part of the station's £1m overhaul, show two kissing silhouettes in a red circle with a red line through them.

And they did not go down well. Especially as they arrived in time for Valentine's Day. Said one commuter, Ruth Hardman: 'I was gobsmacked when I saw the signs. They should spend the money on something more worthwhile.' Another traveller, Peter Kallis commented: 'It's plain daft. I don't see the point of it all. Why bother setting regulations on where people can express their emotions? Whatever happened to acting on impulse? It is the sort of thing you'd expect to see in Nazi Germany under Hitler or in Russia under Stalin.'

Honest student Paul Leicester found a mobile in the street while out celebrating his 18th birthday in April. He handed it in to the police – and was arrested. Unfortunately for Paul, the phone had been reported stolen and he became number one suspect when he presented it to Southport Police Station. He was held for four hours during which he had to empty his pockets, take off his shoes, pose for an incriminating criminal mug shot and provide fingerprints and a DNA swab. No-one, it seemed, was interested in the fact that Paul had even gone to the lengths of trying to let the phone owner know the mobile had been found by calling the last person who had sent a text message to it. Said a rightly miffed Paul: 'The police said the mobile had been reported stolen so I was in possession of stolen goods. What kind of person steals a phone and then hands it in to the police? My parents have brought me up to do the right thing. Being arrested is no way to celebrate your 18th birthday.' Police eventually decided not to proceed with any charges against Paul. Commented a spokesman: 'As a matter of course, we are reviewing the circumstances of the arrest.'

When it was announced in May that stores would have to display signs warning pregnant women that they must not drink and put up posters warning of heart disease and all the other problems associated with alcohol abuse, critics said it was just another example of our nanny state. Especially as the shops would be forced by law to help with the Home Office campaign. The Home Office, in turn, said that the posters were designed to persuade customers to buy and drink less alcohol and were needed because 'there is confusion among the general public' about how much one should drink. The posters would show how much alcohol is contained in the drinks on sale and list recommended daily limits as well as the dangers to health. In the same campaign, pubs were also ordered to list alcohol content and were banned from any promotions encouraging irresponsible drinking. Commented TaxPayers' Alliance spokesman Susie Squire: 'It's common sense that pregnant women should not drink and almost all have done that for centuries. This is yet another example of the nanny state which will cost businesses and the taxpayer yet more money and will patronise responsible customers.' And Tory MP Ann Widdecombe added: 'The idea that people don't already know that binge-drinking and consuming alcohol while pregnant is harmful is ludicrous. It is also more bureaucracy and a complete waste of time and money.'

It was the perfect solution for two working mums. Police officers Lucy Jarrett and Leanne Shepherd, both 32, shared child-minding of their little girls, enabling both of them to carry out their jobs. It was an arrangement that had worked well for two and a half years, with the bonus that Ms Jarrett's little girl Amy, aged 3 and Ms Shepherd's little girl Edie, aged 2, had become the best of friends. Then, in September, it seemed someone 'grassed' on the two detectives from Aylesbury, Buckinghamshire, and the women were labelled as illegal child-minders. Ofsted, the educational monitoring body, judged the arrangement to be illegal because its rules state that adults cannot be rewarded for looking after a child for more than two hours a day outside the child's home. No money ever passed between the two mums of course – but Ofsted said the free child care they benefited from was 'reward' enough. Ms Jarrett and Ms Shepherd were told that if they wished to continue their informal child-minding routine, they would have to register with Ofsted as childminders, undergo criminal record checks, pass a safety inspection and ensure the children in their charge met certain development and educational targets. Further, they were told that they would be subject to impromptu visits if they continued to look after each other's child. The two women, obviously more law-abiding than most, were horrified to learn they were breaking the law and were forced to sign their girls up with a nursery.

But said Ms Jarrett: 'It was the perfect arrangement. We trust each other implicitly. Our children have grown up together. We would both know our children were safe.' The women's plight caused public outrage when it hit the news in September. Margaret Morrissey of the campaign group Parents Outloud said: 'This Big Brother attitude to children and parents has got to stop.' Ofsted said it was simply implementing Labour's 2006 Childcare Act. The Government said it would have a word with Ofsted to ensure a 'common sense and measured approach' to the problem.

Nottingham earned the reputation of a 'no go' area in October after its Labour-run City Council introduced stringent rules that may have been aimed at cleaning it up, but instead resulted in residents feeling authorities were playing dirty with their money. Putting up a missing cat poster on a street sign, leaving an empty wheelie bin in the road, smoking in the wrong place or leaving a car engine running were all announced as offences which could lead to a fine of anything up to £300. Critics of the scheme said it was just another excuse to raise extra cash at a time when the recession was hitting local council revenue from car parking and planning applications. Said one resident, 45-year-old Andrew Shoesmith: 'This has a very totalitarian feel to it. Police and their pretend police friends being able to dish out fines for things that are not crimes is very worrying. If it is a crime to sit in a car with the engine running then this country really has gone mad.' Said another, 29-year-old Anthony Platt: 'Whatever will they find to fine us for next? Looking at people in a strange way? Walking on the cracks in the pavements? Wearing a loud shirt in a built-up area?' Nottingham has 100 uniformed Community Police Protection Officers who work alongside police dealing with anti-social behaviour. The council said the penalties were brought in as a response to public opinion. Supporting punishing offenders, chief anti-social behaviour officer Richard Antcliff remarked: 'When we survey people, the things that trouble them most are not robbery, burglary and other crimes, but the low-level, anti-social rubbish and grime stuff. This will allow us to tackle day-to-day annoyances.' Like Nottingham City Council perhaps?

It was a sad state of affairs when the traditional Scout jamboree came under threat in October after ninety years. The reason? Our ever-growing concern over infiltration by paedophiles – a fear highlighted this year by sickening events at a children's nursery. The annual Scout gathering attracts around 40,000 members from many countries to celebrate the movement's founding by Lord Baden-Powell. But such a large event in Britain calls for thousands of foreign adult volunteers – who, in the current climate, would have to register and undergo a

criminal record check to confirm their suitability to work alongside young people. Volunteers failing to register under the new
Independent Safeguarding Authority face criminal prosecution
and a fine of up to £5,000. But such a stringent check would be
near impossible because of the huge numbers involved. Said
Scout Association spokesman Simon Carter: 'When we hold big
international jamborees we rely on adults from other parts of the
world coming in and staffing these events. The rules for
checking people out suggest that if they are to come along and
do intensive activity they would have to be checked. Clearly we
cannot do that – it's just not possible.' Mr Carter said he believed
adults who are supervised while in contact with children should
be exempt from the new rules. The association wrote to the then
Children's Secretary Ed Balls asking him to allow voluntary
groups greater flexibility and warning that parents wanting to
volunteer for such groups would be deterred by the ISA's
'bureaucratic and difficult' regulations. Said a spokesman for the
department for Children, Schools and Families: 'We recognise
the importance of children attending and participating in international events such as jamborees organised by the Scout
Association and would not wish the vetting and barring scheme
to act as a deterrent to them going ahead. While the fine detail is
yet to be finalised, we are working in collaboration with the
Scout Association and others to ensure that the practical
operation of the scheme does not impede the operation of these
events.'

The creation of the ISA was announced in September 2009
amid great controversy. It was estimated that around one in four
adults could eventually be registered with the scheme and that
every doctor, nurse, prison officer and school governor was
among those who would have to undergo clearance.

West Yorkshire farmer 65-year-old Ronald Norcliffe should
have been relieved when Government officials gave a tubercu-
losis all-clear to his livestock. Instead, he got himself into a bit of
a barn-ey with the representatives of the Kirklees environmental

health department and the Department for Environment, Food and Rural Affairs (DEFRA). For when the inspectors asked Mr Norcliffe where he kept his cattle in winter and were told in a barn underneath his house, they virtually 'did' him for cruelty to cows. The accommodation was declared unsuitable because it did not have an electric light and because the barn doors were kept closed (because, explained Mr Norcliffe, he wanted to keep his cows warm). The little farm at Scammonden then became the focus of rather eccentric concern considering Mr Norcliffe had managed to run it quite happily for thirty years without outside help. First he was served with an 'improvement notice' and then followed three official visits before he was finally charged with 'failing to meet the psychological and ethological needs' of a cow. Note the singular, here. For Mr Norcliffe has just the one cow and calf at his farm. He was fined £150 in October by Huddersfield magistrates for his 'crime' – for which the maximum punishment is nearly a year in prison. He was also ordered to pay £50 costs plus a £15 'victim surcharge'. Prosecuting, Carol English told the court: 'The defendant had been given four warnings, received visits and been given advice, but despite all the help and assistance, he has failed to provide adequate lighting.' The farmer didn't actually have electricity at his smallholding but had offered to provide light in the barn with a generator. Mr Norcliffe's lawyer, Bob Carr, quite under-standably admitted to not knowing exactly what the 'psychological and ethological needs' of the cows are, adding: 'I'm sure Mr Norcliffe doesn't either. I still have no idea how much lighting is appropriate for a cow.'

Oh, for the days when a village bobby could clip a teenage wrong-doer around the ear and everyone felt justice was done . . . not nowadays. And particularly not if you are a member of the public who is fed up with hooligans throwing stones at your windows. Disabled pensioner, 71-year-old Renate Bowling, took to her walking frame and went outside her house in Thornton Cleveleys, Lancs, to confront a 17-year-old youth after catching him mid stone-throwing. The confrontation culminated in Mrs Bowling poking him in the chest. The teenage terror complained to police that he had been assaulted. Mrs Bowling's version was different. She claimed he had hold of her wrists and bruised them and had 'the gall to call it self-defence', adding: 'The police put me in the back of their van like a sack of spuds and took me to the station where they questioned me. Then a few days later I was told I was being prosecuted. I could not believe it, neither could my family.' German-born Mrs Bowling is a survivor of World War II who endured some time in East Berlin before marrying an Englishman and settling in Britain. She later appeared at Blackpool Magistrates Court, was given a conditional discharge for six months and ordered to pay £50 costs. Julie Reilly, prosecuting, told magistrates: 'This defendant says he was playing football in the street when there was an incident between himself and the defendant. Had the defendant accepted her criminality in prodding the aggrieved in the chest there and then, this could well have been dealt with in a different way.' Originally Mrs Bowling had intended to deny the offence but after a long deliberation between the Crown Prosecution Service and her defence, Mrs Bowling admitted the charge of assault. She retorted after the court case: 'What justice is there? There are a group of youths who throw gravel at my window and use foul language against me. I saw one of them throw the stones against my window from my bedroom. I went out and found him hiding behind a wall. I poked my finger out at him and told him what I thought of him. He called me "some ****ing German woman". Then the police arrested me – I thought "What a joke. What is going on?" I had to borrow £20 from a friend to pay the court costs as I only had £30 on me. It has all been a nightmare.' Nigel Beeson who defended Mrs Bowling in court commented: 'This is a very sad case for those concerned – a 71-year-old granny charged with assaulting a 17-year-old boy. It was a prod, there were no injuries.' One assumes the lad received no official admonishment at all.

*   *   *

A young church-going mother who told off her 11-year-old son and 4-year-old daughter after they behaved badly at a supermarket in Southampton, Hants, was not only followed home by an off-duty police officer and questioned by two on-duty ones, but was reported to Southampton City Council's Children's Services who sent her a letter reporting that the 'chastisement' of her children in a public place was now 'on record'. It was all very distressing for the 34-year-old mum (who quite rightly wanted to remain anonymous) who, like many others, had simply been frustrated when what should have been a good summer's day turned out to be bad weather – and the children were a bit stir-crazy because they could not play outdoors. Admitting she had threatened to give the children a hiding after they ran a little wild in the shop and were quarrelling between themselves, the woman, a bookshop manager said: 'I have never been in trouble with the police before and I have great respect for them, so I was absolutely shocked. When they told me about the off-duty police officer, I couldn't believe it. He must have only seen the end part of a long day where they had played up and slid on the floors in the supermarket.' The woman felt she had been the focus of attention because in her admonishment of the children, she alluded to smacking the boy earlier in the day when he had misbehaved, but said it was rare for her to treat either of her children that way. The Children's Services Department said it would take no further action but that the incident would remain on file, stating: 'It is very important that we keep records of any concerns raised to us about children in the city.' And a spokesman for Hampshire Police said that the off-duty officer felt 'it was not an ordinary telling-off and because of what the woman said and the way her children reacted to it, it gave our officer reasonable grounds for concern'.

The Green New Deal called for by the Environment Agency may have been aimed at reducing global warming but it left everyone from motorists to householders and holidaymakers feeling very hot under the collar. For the Agency was pushing for a 'carbon tax' – meaning we would all be given a personal allowance which would be reduced if we used our car, turned up our heating or took too many flights. If the allowance is used up, then we would have to pay for more credits. Luckily, the plan would not be fully operational for twenty years or so, giving us time to dwell on it. But opposers said it was an 'Orwellian' scheme restricting the individual's freedom to choose how they conduct their lives as well as destined to cripple businesses. Commented economist Ruth Lea: 'This is getting beyond a joke. This is all about the control of the individual and you begin to wonder whether this is what the green agenda has always been about.' Supporting the plans, unveiled in November 2009, a spokesman for the Environment Agency said: 'A lot of people who do cycling will get money back. It will probably only be bankers and those on extravagant lifestyles who would lose out.'

When pregnant Mary Cooke called the police after nearly being knocked off her feet by a speeding car she ended up with her home being under investigation. For the 27-year-old mother-to-be and her husband Peter were in the middle of decorating their semi-detached house in Newcastle-under-Lyme, Staffs, in preparation for the new arrival. But police took one look at the wallpaper hanging off the walls and the general mid-decorating mess, and reported the couple to social services because they felt the home environment was not suitable for a child. Mrs Cooke then received a letter from Staffordshire County Council which she said was expressing fears for the safety of her baby. Said Mrs Cooke: 'I admit the house was in a bit of a state when the police called, but we were in the middle of wallpapering to make sure everything was nice for when the baby arrives. The letter made me feel sick. I cannot believe I have been unjustly branded in this way.' A Staffordshire Police spokesman justified the female officer's actions by saying: 'Our officers aim to act in the best interests of everyone they come into contact with. Their role involves liaising with colleagues from partner agencies on a regular basis.' The council stated that it was 'looking into the matter with the co-operation of the person concerned'.

Employees of multi-million pound meat-supplying company Dunbia did not mince words when the Ulster-based firm insisted they clocked on and off every time they took a toilet break. In short, spending a penny costs some of them as much as £30 a week under this system because their pay is docked for each visit. It all seems rather a load of bull for the meat company that has an annual turnover of £450 million. A group of employees from Dunbia's eleven factories in Ireland and the UK complained and their union, Unite, became involved. Said regional officer Cathy Rudderforth: 'Dunbia is making money every time a worker visits the loo and that money is coming out of the workers' wage packets. It's outrageous that in 2009 workers have to endure the indignity of clocking out for toilet breaks.' One former employee claimed he had been sacked for challenging the orders. A spokesman for Dunbia said the system was introduced on health and safety grounds and that employees were simply required to clock in and out of food-processing areas. It was a practice that had been running satisfactorily for five years and that to ensure employees do not suffer 'financial disadvantage' their weekly wages are increased to compensate for toilet breaks.

It was a rather more sophisticated step up from the twitching of net curtains to see what your neighbours are up to . . . the installation of £1,000 CCTV cameras in homes to monitor what was going on in the streets outside. In a real Big Brother scenario, each camera was linked to a laptop computer and was accessible online by police and council officials twenty-four hours a day. Those in favour of the scheme, tested by Croydon Council in south London, said it would help identify anyone causing anti-social behaviour and mean a speedy prosecution. Critics, however, said it was just another measure in the ever-increasing sinister Big Brother surveillance that Britain was encompassing.

Commented Alex Deane, director of the TaxPayers' Alliance Big Brother Watch (yes, there really is one!): 'People accept these cameras into their homes because they are afraid. The council might be installing them with the best intentions but the end result is a culture of fear and mistrust driven by a failure by the borough and the police to have proper law enforcement in this area.' Simon Davies of Privacy International added: 'It shows we have become a Britain obsessed with CCTV. Unless the public are aware of where these cameras are, I believe this council should be taken to court for a breach of human rights.' Local councillor Gavin Barwell denied the cameras would be used to spy on neighbours, stating: 'No-one should have to put up with anti-social behaviour on their doorstep and these cameras give us another means of responding quickly if it occurs.' If the cameras proved a success, more would be installed . . .

The snooping into our privacy continued when it was announced that same month that Health and Safety inspectors could be given unprecedented access to monitor homes where children are considered to be at the greatest risk of 'unintentional injury'. Safety devices such as smoke alarms, stair gates and window locks would then be fitted where necessary by council staff, and GPs and midwives would be encouraged to report any safety worries they have when making routine visits to homes where there are children. Of course, any measures which protect babies, children and young children are commendable (especially in the light of so many Social Service inadequacies) but in this case, some felt it constituted intrusion. London GP and head of the British Medical Association's GP committee, Dr Laurence Buckman agreed that 'dangerous homes' should be identified, but added: 'These proposals are very intrusive and parents would be very angry with me if they invited me into their home and I reported them to a third party. That's not my job and it would mess up my relationship with patients.' Dr Buckman did, of course, reiterate a doctor's obligation to report any fears that a child is being abused to social services. The measures were drawn up by the National Institute for Health and Clinical Medicine and labelled by critics as a 'waste of money, but worse than that, an abuse of power', with the accusation that it was all 'another extension of the state's invasive powers to poke their noses into people's private lives and nanny people. People have enough of a job paying their bills and keeping a roof over their heads without having to worry about inspectors knocking and scoring them on how competent they are at running their own home . . .'

Parents were given no let-up when again, that same month, it was announced that the Department of Health wanted all families in England and Wales to fill out 83-point questionnaires before their 5-year-olds started school. The forms asked very intrusive questions such as 'How does your child behave when you leave the room?' and if a child had been known to steal, lie or cheat. There are also questions about a child's eating habits, exercise and friends. The information will be held indefinitely on NHS databases and although described as 'confidential' will be used by health workers in cases where support is thought to be needed. The nationwide questionnaires – called School Entry Wellbeing Review Forms – were decided upon following a trial of families in Lincolnshire as part of a 'Healthy Child Programme'. The DoH said it needed to build up a detailed picture of families and children's development. Children will fill in the questionnaires themselves when they are old enough. Dylan Sharpe of the Big Brother Watch pressure group commented: 'This is incredibly intrusive and asks questions which, quite frankly, Lincolnshire Community Health Services do not need to know and have no right knowing. Even worse, the NHS Trust has failed to make it clear that this is a voluntary questionnaire. I would advise any parent receiving it to stick it straight in the bin.' Parents are not legally bound to fill in the forms but if they don't they are likely to be visited by community nurses whose role is to identify vulnerable families. The Department of Health issued a statement: 'Many local areas currently administer a questionnaire to parents as a basis for a review at school entry. The Healthy Child Programme included the commitment to build on good practice to make available a standardised evaluated version. We will ensure this complies with legal requirements in relation to data-handling and approaches to encourage take-up. This questionnaire will be an additional tool to safeguard and support all children's health and wellbeing.'

The year ended with a real 'super snooper' revelation – that there could be as many as 20,000 officials legally entitled to enter our homes without warning, consent, a warrant or a policeman in tow to supervise. The 'powers of entry' legislation was set out by the Home Office (the existing Labour Government got the blame) and allowed for an average of forty-seven officials within every local authority to knock on our doors and quite legitimately make a nuisance of themselves. Reasons for the intrusion are ludicrous and included: inspecting a property to ensure illegal or unregulated hypnotism is not taking place (Hypnotism Act 1952); powers to inspect for the presence of rabbits (Pest Act 1954); to check the energy ratings on refrigerators (Energy Information Refrigerators regulations 2004) and to see if pot plants have plant pests or do not have a 'plant passport' (Plant Health Order 2005).

In all, there are over 1,000 laws in place permitting an 'official' to enter your home. The research was carried out by privacy campaigners, the Big Brother Watch group which found that nationwide there were at least 14,793 official snoopers who are often untraceable on a council's website and who may be unvetted and inadequately trained for the job. There were also openings for abuse of power and downright rudeness to unsuspecting householders who have the misfortune to answer the door to one of these snoopers. Even more sinister was the fact that some councils such as Manchester City Council, Sheffield City Council and Sunderland City Council refused to supply information to Big Brother Watch leading to speculation that the official snoopers could top 20,000. Who has the highest number of these dodgy employees? Topping the list is Northamptonshire County Council with 499 officers, followed by Glasgow City Council with 483 and Conwy County Borough Council with 361. Defending the rather chilling situation, a Government spokesman said: 'It's vital that we strike the right balance between privacy and security and that is why the Government is clear these powers should only be used when they are necessary and proportionate. Power of entry should exist only where strict criteria are met.' This will not satisfy law-abiding citizens of course. And, added Alex Deane, director of the Big Brother Watch: 'Once a man's home was his castle. Today the Big Brother state wants to inspect, regulate and standardise the inside of our homes.'

That same month, it was also revealed that there are now 60,000 council-snooping cameras trained on the public – three times that of ten years ago and one for every 1,000 of the UK's population. That number does not include the thousands that are used by private companies and central Government – said to be around a staggering 4 million CCTVs in all. But do they catch the bad guys? Well, no, it seems not. For despite claims that the cameras are an 'important tool' in crime-fighting, often the filming is so poor that culprits cannot be identified. This does not stop hapless motorists being filmed then fined for using bus lanes, however. A Local Government Association spokesman vehemently defended the use of closed circuit television, stating it was their existence that brought London's infamous 'July 21 would-be bombers' to justice and that 'in tough financial times, councils are not going to spend money on installing CCTV cameras unless they genuinely believe doing so will help reduce crime, catch criminals and make people feel safer'. At least £170m in Home Office grants has been spent on installing the council cameras. The massive rise in CCTVs was revealed by Big Brother Watch using the Freedom of Information access. Commented Alex Deane: 'The quality of footage is frequently too poor to be used in courts, the cameras are often turned off to

QUANGO CRACKERS

We have basically had enough . . . especially knowing that we also have to contend with 1,162 'Quango' groups employing 700,000 staff and all either giving us useless information or telling us how to run our lives. Top of the crop was the British Potato Council with a staff of fifty and raising its £6m a year running costs with a surcharge on every sack of potatoes we buy. (The Council tells us to eat more potatoes while the Food Standards Agency tells us not to!) Another group, Partnership UK, gives chief executive James Stewart a deal worth £505,000 for his job to 'support and accelerate delivery of infrastructure renewal, high quality public services and the efficient use of public assets through better and stronger partnerships between the public and private sectors'. The £38m watchdog quango the Tenant Services Authority resolved just twelve complaints in its first year while the remaining 396 were passed on to other organisations. And English Heritage, which manages more than 400 ancient monuments, failed to meet its targets of increasing the number of ethnic minorities, disabled and poor people to its historic sites. English Heritage was set the 'diversity' targets in 2005 by the Government as a condition of its £250 million a year budget. But Edward Leigh, Conservative chairman of the Commons public accounts committee said the targets were unrealistic and that neither ministers nor officials at the Department for Culture, Media and Sport seemed to have any idea how to achieve them. He said: 'The proportion of the UK population visiting historic sites is already some 70 per cent, an impressive total, and most of the people who don't visit say they are not interested in doing so. It is hard to see what useful purpose was achieved by setting targets to increase visits from this or that under-represented group.'

In January 2010 we heard how energy companies were bombarding households with 200 million free eco-light bulbs even though we didn't really need them. One supplier, npower, sent out 12 million over Christmas – which must have delighted postmen – prompting a Government ban on the mail-out from

January 1. The company faced a £40 million fine if it failed to meet its energy-saving targets but denied it was cluttering up our homes with unwanted bulbs. A spokesman said: 'We want to make sure that npower customers don't miss out on a simple way to save energy and reduce their bills. We're spending more than £350 million on our energy-saving programmes and free light bulbs are only a tiny part of this.'

The free lightbulb scheme – paid for by householders through fuel bills with an average gas and electricity customer paying £38 a year towards subsidies for green projects according to energy watchdog group Ofgem – allowed suppliers to meet their legally binding targets for improving home energy efficiency. Companies began the light bulb bombardment in 2008 after ministers ordered them to invest in projects to improve home energy efficiency as part of a Government scheme designed to cut carbon emissions. The suppliers were allowed to choose their measures which included subsidised loft insulation, but realised the cheapest way of meeting targets was to use the postal service to send out free light bulbs. They could send up to two to each household without having to prove they were used, needed or even wanted. The Department for Energy and Climate Change announced it would ban unsolicited eco-bulbs because too many were left unused. A report stated: 'Government is increasingly concerned that the number of bulbs already distributed has been so high that it may work out at more than the average number of highest-use light fittings in a house. As such, there is an increasing risk to carbon savings under the scheme where bulbs are not used, are installed in low-use light fittings or replace existing low-energy bulbs.'

Naturally, there are many who think quangos are a waste of time, resources and the tax-payers' money. Said Andrew Haldenby of the group Reform: 'Boil down everything wrong with British Government and you get a quango, they should be abolished.' Susie Squire of the TaxPayers' Alliance was even more critical of the quango waste, saying: 'Our quango state is bloated, inefficient and unaccountable. These bodies need to justify their existence and earn their keep – or face the axe.'

save money and control rooms are rarely manned twenty-four hours a day. We should all feel safer with more police on the beat, there would be fewer crimes and those crimes that do occur would be solved faster.' The group said it believed CCTV is there only to appease neighbourhoods suffering from anti-social behaviour problems. Over to Mike Milks, chief executive of Scyron which helps police analyse CCTV images, who said: 'We estimate that about half of the CCTV cameras in the country are next to useless when it comes to safeguarding the public against crime and assisting the police to secure convictions.'

January 2010 saw the end of a police case against a man accused of sending an offensive email – even though they had the wrong person. The 45-year-old IT boss, who asked not to be named throughout his ordeal, was arrested in front of his wife and young son at home in August 2009. He was handcuffed, ordered to accompany police officers to the station, spent four hours in a cell and even had his DNA taken – together with his computer and other internet equipment. It was then discovered that the email was not sent by him but by a colleague, 39-year-old Paul Osmond – who was also arrested but finally told there would be no further police action. The email concerned related to a planning appeal by a gypsy and was deemed offensive because it stated 'It's the "do as you likey attitude" that I am against' – with the word 'likey' rhyming with the derogatory term for gypsy, 'pikey'. The email was sent by the colleague from the businessman's company to a website at Rother District Council, East Sussex, on which members of the public can comment on planning applications. Commented the company owner after his ordeal: 'I was extremely angry. I was relaxing in the comfort of my home on a Sunday afternoon and then I was in a police car under arrest – all for an innocent comment by a colleague. I have never had any criminal record and try my best to teach my children right from wrong. This was a ridiculously heavy-handed police reaction to what they perceived as a racist comment. I am not in the least bit racist and neither is Paul Osmond. The gypsy family concerned did not complain.' The appeal centred on keeping a mobile home in an area declared as one of outstanding beauty overlooking the Battle of Hastings site. Mr Osmond, quite rightly too, was also not happy being arrested. He said: 'I made it clear to the police that I am absolutely not racist. I said I was simply registering my objection to this application because it is 200ft from the most important and historical battlefield in the country. I now feel I am not even able to express an opinion for fear of being arrested by police. One of my closest friends is an Irish traveller and he uses the term "pikey" all the time. This is the ultimate in political correctness going off the scale.' Sussex Police said they had arrested the company boss on 'suspicion of committing a racial or religious-aggravated offence' with Chief Inspector Heather Keating adding: 'Sussex Police have a legal duty to promote community cohesion and tackle unlawful discrimination. We are satisfied we acted appropriately in identifying the computer used and through this, the identity of the writer of the offending line.' The local council felt it had done the right thing too, with a spokesman explaining: 'As far as we are concerned it was an offensive comment so we got in touch with the police.' It still seems rather unfair that as a result of all this, the businessman has to accept that his DNA – taken from an innocent man – will now remain indefinitely on the police database.

The whole DNA issue was highlighted when it emerged that for every innocent person removed from the DNA database a further 250 are added. In November 2008 the European Court ruled that it was unlawful to indefinitely store DNA samples from people who were later cleared. But since then, only 400 people had successfully appealed to police to have that done – with 487,000 being added, of whom around 101,000 were estimated to be entirely innocent. The figures were discovered by Liberal Democratic Cabinet Office spokesman Jenny Willott who said: 'It is appalling that the Government has taken the DNA of 100,000 innocent people since they were told the practice is illegal. Despite the Government's promises to abide by the European Court ruling, they are still doing everything they can to avoid it.' Chief Constable of West Midlands Police, Sir Paul Scott-Lee said DNA matches from the database solve only one crime in 150. But a Home Office spokesman insisted: 'It is crucial that we do everything we can to protect the public by preventing crime and bringing offenders to justice.'

This line was reinforced when we learned in February 2010 that detectives were ordering weekly searches of the national DNA database for people with no immediate connection to any crime! *The Mail on Sunday* obtained figures which showed that police searched the DNA records for innocent people 363 times in six years. The searches are used when crime scene DNA samples produce no direct match on the system. Investigators then trawl millions of other records looking for a partial match which might indicate the suspect is related to an innocent person on the system. As the newspaper pointed out, these 'familial DNA searches' raised new questions about the increasing number of innocent people's records being held on the DNA register because 'a partial match could lead to police launching a background investigation and even a surveillance operation, targeting an innocent person while searching for a family member'. Opposers to this approach of tracking down criminals while involving the innocent said that only convicted criminals should have their DNA kept on the register. Commented Helen Wallace of GeneWatch: 'This should never be used as a routine technique and there should be far more transparency and over-sight about when and where the police are ordering these kind of searches. We have no objection to its use in investigating serious unsolved crimes but the guidelines for its use have never been published so we have no idea where the police draw the line. There is a real danger of mission creep. We need to know when and where these searches are being used and its use needs to be severely restricted.' There were great concerns over data protection and human rights. Quite rightly so. For nearly a million people – including children – who have never been convicted of a crime were still kept on the National DNA Database despite the understanding they would be destroyed in response to the ruling by the European Court of Human Rights. The Court ruled that 'blanket retention of suspects' was unlawful. To balance the argument, it must be said that several criminals have been convicted using the 'familial DNA searches'. In 2004 a Surrey man was convicted of manslaughter after he was linked to a crime scene through a close relative's DNA profile. The National Policing Improvement Agency said that seventy-three similar searches in the last two years demonstrated it was not routinely used, had to be approved by a high-ranking officer and in 'the most serious crime investigations only'. The Home Office introduced a ruling to offer some reassurance about the whole DNA/innocent people problem. It recommended a six-year limit on keeping DNA of most unconvicted adults and 16 to 17-year-olds. Unconvicted children under 16 would face a three-year limit. Repeat offenders and those convicted of serious crimes have their DNA profiles held indefinitely.

In yet another hair-raising example of hysterical health and safety laws, barber Lee Haynes was fined £450 on December 7th 2009, for illegally disposing of waste from his shop. He was guilty of failing to provide waste transfer notes in respect of AFH Ladies Hair Design in Sudbury, Suffolk . . . He also owns Lee's Barber Shop next door. His crime? Bagging up hair clippings and leaving them on a skip. Apparently members of the public had complained. Babergh District Council decided that although the clippings were not 'dangerous', peroxide and dyes which might be found on the hair were potentially harmful to the general public. Officials staked out Mr Haynes' premises, took photographs, raided the two shops and then prosecuted him under the Environmental Protection Act 1990. It turns out that nowadays any hairdresser wanting to dispose of clippings must apply for special permission and have them collected by an authorised agent at a cost of £300 a year. The barber commented:

'I thought it was a wind-up when I got a phone call and they said they were involved in a police anti-terrorism check. They wanted to know how much peroxide I had got on the premises and whether it was kept under lock and key. We hardly use the stuff here but I was told that unless I gave full details they would send an officer round to check.'

Mr Haynes was not present at the hearing at Bury St Edmunds Magistrates Court and found guilty in his absence. As well as the fine, he was ordered to pay £300 prosecution costs and a 'victim' surcharge of £15. At an earlier hearing in September that year, Mr Haynes was also found guilty of failing to provide waste transfer notes for his barber shop and was ordered to pay a £200 fine and £300 costs. James Buckingham, Babergh's Principal Environmental Protection Officer said the prosecution of Mr Haynes was taken as a last resort and that the council endeavoured to work with local businesses to help them comply with the law. Mr Buckingham added: 'Babergh officers did their utmost to assist Mr Haynes in order to ensure he was disposing of his waste correctly and maintaining the correct paperwork. Advisory letters, in-person visits, formal interview requests, as well as the opportunity to take a Fixed Penalty Notice instead of legal action were ignored . . . Businesses are duty-bound by law to store commercial waste safely and securely and only pass it on to someone else with the authority to dispose of it correctly. Waste transfer notes are needed to record that this is being done and Mr Haynes was unable to provide them.' Hairdressing waste, said Mr Buckingham, can contain hazardous chemicals such as bleach powder, hydrogen peroxide and acidic or alkaline perm solutions.

It was reported in January 2010 that taxmen were increasingly using anti-terror laws to snoop on those suspected of minor breaches of the rules. Usage of the laws had risen by 75 per cent in the last four years and in one year alone, 2009, officials at Revenue and Customs began more than 5,600 investigations which relied on the Labour Government's controversial surveillance laws. The Regulation of Investigatory Powers Act allows public sector officials to watch or follow individuals and use spies to inform on them. The Revenue claimed that the powers are only used in cases where people are suspected of importing drugs, arms and other contraband or in major VAT fraud investigations. But there have been cases of suggested misuse of the powers with taxmen snooping on tax-payers and small businesses, a couple who were spied on over suspicions they were cheating on school catchment area rules and people being followed for littering or allowing their dog to foul public places. Commented Conservative communities spokesman Caroline Spelman: 'We already know that Labour's tax inspectors are spying on family homes to prepare for a painful council tax revaluation. Now it is clear that the tax officials are using anti-terror powers to spy on the personal tax affairs of hard-working families anything up to fifteen times a day. Labour's surveillance laws are routinely being abused and over-used by town hall officials and quangos and turning Britain into a Stasi state.' A spokesman for Revenue and Customs said that the body works within 'the established safeguards when using the powers granted under RIPA' and that it 'properly addresses the requirements of both necessity and proportionality. No allegations about HMRC potential misuse of RIPA have been upheld.'

In January 2009 it was the School Entry Wellbeing Review Forms quizzing little children on various subjects such as if they had ever lied and what they ate. Exactly a year later, Big Brother struck again in a similar way. The 'lifestyle' quizzes, backed by the Department of Health, were piloted in Erewash, Derbyshire, where primary school pupils as young as 5 filled in the forms at 'healthy eating' after-school clubs to which parents were invited. The children were asked to colour in answers to questions – for example, the amount of fruit they ate each day from a selection of pictures of fruit – compared to their consumption of crisps and fizzy drinks. They were also asked about their TV-watching habits, family time, if they ate breakfast, how they got to school and even if they 'like themselves' (answered by ticking a thumbs up or thumbs down sign). Although the survey was not compulsory, the children were strongly encouraged to complete it. Slightly older children aged 7 were given an even more detailed quiz asking such questions as how many hours they spent playing computer games. Results are stored on a database allowing families considered to be 'at risk' to be referred to doctors or social services. A spokesman for Erewash council said the questions followed the guidelines set by NICE, the NHS's regulatory body and added: 'They will help us target families at risk of obesity. We can encourage parents to attend sessions with social services or GPs.' Following the trial at Erewash, the questionnaires were sent out to 200 other schools nationwide with interest shown by other councils. Privacy campaigners were not altogether comfortable. Said Alex Deane of Big Brother Watch: 'The State does not bring up children, parents do. There is an important distinction between teaching and nannying – or even bullying – and this oversteps the mark.' Civil Liberties campaigner Josie Appleton added: 'Councils and schools should concentrate on providing everyone with a good education. But they should keep their noses out of children's lunchboxes and away from the family dinner table.'

Britain's second largest power supplier, Scottish and Southern Energy, was accused of introducing a 'draconian' health and safety regime which would see any of its 20,000 employees facing disciplinary action if they failed to comply. There were 'Five Safety Golden Rules: Reverse Park, Wear Personal Protective Equipment, Assess Risks, Hold Handrails and Accept Challenges.' Said one SSE employee: 'The dos and don'ts are becoming so ridiculous they are losing their effect. Staff feel the measures are so draconian that they can barely move around the workplace without breaking a Golden Rule. Under current company policy, anyone seen using stairs without holding the handrail must accept a "challenge" from a colleague or manager. It's known as a "yellow card". If you are a repeat offender then the company can begin disciplinary action.' SSE confirmed that if a worker continually refused to respond to such challenges the issue would be raised with their boss. Said a spokesman: 'Reversing into a static parking bay is safer than reversing out into a road or car park which may have traffic and pedestrian movement which you cannot easily see. A quick internal search will highlight the number of fatalities each year arising from people falling down stairs. If everyone held the handrail when going up and down stairs it might not prevent all deaths but it would probably prevent many of them.'

It was back to bureaucratic and bothersome Big Brother bin business in February 2010 when it was announced that an army of 'bin police' was primed to check the rubbish of millions of families in Britain with dawn squads swooping to expose house-holders who are not recycling their refuse. Pilot schemes each costing around £10,000 had been instigated in parts of Dorset, London, Suffolk and Shropshire – where Shropshire Council admitted an independent research company had been employed to collect rubbish from a sample of homes. This Zero Waste Places Scheme was launched by Environment Secretary Hilary Benn with the idea that people have several recycling bins including a slop bucket for food waste and bins for glass, plastic, cardboard, paper, tins and garden waste. Everything that could be burned, re-used, recycled or left to rot needed to be sorted and collected, with a traditional black bin to be used for what should be a very small amount of rubbish left over to go to a traditional landfill site. Laws passed in 2005 give town halls power to enter premises 'to examine and investigate as required' and to 'take samples of articles or substances found, if they think householders have broken any waste rules'. Those who did faced big fines. It was no wonder some critics nicknamed the rubbish crackdown as the 'Talibin' and said it was yet another blow to civil liberties. Bob Neill, Shadow Minister for Local Government said: 'Sinister laws passed by the Government allow inspectors to enter your home and garden, inspect your bins and take away samples and then fine you for breaching minor rules. This Binquisition is another sign of how Labour don't care about the privacy of law-abiding citizens and treat home-owners like common criminals.' Added Doretta Cocks, founder of the Campaign for Weekly Bin Collections: 'The Government must be deluded if it thinks we can achieve zero waste. It is totally unachievable. Having bin police snooping around in dawn raids to take samples of people's bins for analysis is a step too far.'

. . . Could it get worse? Well yes. Britain's bureaucratic blitz on bins was big news again in March that year. And again, it made front page news with the *Daily Mail* announcing: 'Spy chips hidden in 2.5 million dustbins' – '60pc rise in electronic bugs as council snoopers plan pay-as-you-throw tax.' The microchips are fitted to wheelie bins to weigh their contents and families who put out more rubbish pay higher taxes to their local council. The news followed Bristol City's introduction of a 'bin tax' which it claimed was a scheme rewarding those who recycled their waste with cash payments to households who discarded less rubbish. The idea had always been a controversial one. Prime Minister Gordon Brown had promised to drop it in 2008 (but later that year nearly 100 councils ran investigations into the contents of householders' bins; either to check on what rubbish was being dumped or to obtain information on incomes and lifestyles). In January 2009 ministers had to admit the fact that not a single council had applied to try out the pay-as-you-go scheme. In March that year a survey based on Freedom of Information inquiries showed there were forty-two councils using bins with microchips. One year on and similar FOI research revealed there were now sixty-eight – one in five of those councils that collect household rubbish. Responses from councils revealed that 2,629,052 homes had the 'chip and bin' scheme. And it had all seemed to happen so stealthily – despite councils' reluctance to openly join in the 'pay-as-you-throw' tax schemes. Said Alex Deane of Big Brother Watch: 'Councils are waiting until the public aren't watching to begin surveillance on our waste habits, intruding into people's private lives and introducing punitive taxes on what we throw away. The British public doesn't want this technology, these fines or this intrusion. If local authorities have no intention to monitor our waste then they should end the surreptitious installation of these bin microchips.' The Local Government Association claimed microchips were used to improve services to the public with a spokesman commenting: 'Microchips simply identify the house to which a bin belongs. They do not mean councils can analyse what people are throwing away or issue fines . . . if an elderly resident needs help getting their bin collected and returned, a microchip quickly flags it up to the refuse collector, saving time and money.' A microchip could also be used in conjunction with technology on a dustcart too, however – weighing a bin's contents. The Department for Environment, Food and Rural Affairs reinforced the claim that there were no Government plans to bring in microchipped bins and that it was all down to individual local councils. The DEFRA spokesman added: 'Some councils use them to monitor levels of waste. This is not about spying on people or fining them . . .'

West Midlands Police were told not to pursue criminals if they were at the end of the shift in a bid to cut overtime payments. It was answering a police emergency call of its own with British forces under pressure to slash the yearly £500 million overtime budget. The force was the first to undertake the initiative and details of it were contained in an overtime rule book published by the Home Office in March 2010. The book revealed that the force had indeed saved money. ' . . . within 24/7 response, sergeants were clear that officers should finish their work before rest days and not chase detections towards the end of their shift.' Said a spokesman for West Midlands Police: 'Rather than them staying over on overtime to finalise cases and claim detection, they were encouraged to hand over paperwork/prisoners to colleagues to finalise the process, thereby cutting down on overtime. This is not a new practice. We constantly remind officers of the most practical and cost-effective way of dealing with prisoners in order to make the best use of tax-payers' money.' But Paul McKeever, chairman of the Police Federation of England and Wales said the initiative jeopardised public safety, adding: 'I appreciate that in tough economic times there is a need for belts to tighten and for careful consideration to be given on how resources and budgets are allocated. But equally important is ensuring that no squeeze on public funds is ever detrimental to the ability of forces to provide a consistent and effective front-line response. We don't do overtime out of choice, but out of a duty to uphold the law. We cannot just walk away from criminals or turn our back on crimes being committed.'

Like most aspects of our Fool Britannia country, none of it made much sense anyway. For earlier that same month we learned that police officers were being paid hundreds of pounds in overtime for answering the telephone once their shift had finished – with officers entitled to a minimum four hours' pay at a rate of time-and-a-third for just picking up the phone and making a decision while off duty.

Auctioneer 57-year-old Jim Railton could have cracked under the strain when he was charged under the 1981 Wildlife and Countryside Act of offering wild birds' eggs for sale. For the eggs were 100 years old and contained in an Edwardian oak cabinet found by someone clearing out their garage and then offered up for sale at a guide price of £30 to £40 by Mr Railton at a saleroom in Alnwick, Northumberland. But the item and its eggs were spotted in the auction brochure and police raided the sale room after a tip-off from the Royal Society for the Protection of Birds. Under the 1981 Act it is illegal to offer wild birds' eggs for sale, no matter how old they are. The legislation was intended to quite rightly protect endangered bird species from thieves and rogue collectors. Mr Railton, of course, fits into neither of those categories but he was still arrested, taken to Berwick police station, questioned for an hour about where the eggs (all from some of Britain's most common bird species) came from and had his fingerprints and DNA swabs taken. As a former RSPB member, the irony was not lost on him.

He said: 'It must have cost thousands of pounds, and all they needed to do was point out that I shouldn't be selling eggs.' The man who originally found the cabinet in his garage was also interviewed by police twice but not charged. At the time, Northumbria Police confirmed they had charged Mr Railton with 'exposing and advertising for sale a collection of wild birds' eggs'. Alex Deane, director of campaign group Big Brother Watch, was a bit shell-shocked too, saying: 'The RSPB and Northumbria Police should be ashamed of themselves. Jim is a law-abiding man whose life and business have been disrupted. They could have approached this case in a more commonsense way.'

On March 31st, Mr Railton was fined £1,000 and ordered to pay £70 costs and a £15 victim's surcharge after appearing at Alnwick Magistrates Court. He was told: 'Ignorance of the law is no defence.'

Mr Railton admitted the offence but said outside court: 'I am amazed. To give me a criminal record on the basis of what I have done is inequitable. This is more Big Brother.'

4

Driving Us Round the Bend

It was just a moment of frustration but it landed disabled war hero Nassir Abaid Khan with a littering charge. Soldier Mr Khan, 44, who served with the SAS during the 1990–1991 Gulf War, was given a parking ticket for leaving his car outside a barber's shop in Blackburn, Lancashire. Realising he had forgotten to display his disabled driver's badge, he tried to remonstrate with parking attendant Sharon Wallbank. He showed her his disabled sticker but she refused to cancel the ticket. In a flash of fury, Mr Khan tried to stick the parking ticket on Ms Wallbank's jacket but it fell to the floor. Mr Khan immediately picked it up, took it to the town hall and had it cancelled. But two weeks later he got a notice in the post accusing him of littering. Mr Khan, showing the true grit that awarded him three service medals and a special commendation for his bravery in the first Gulf War before an accident in training which broke his back, decided to fight the case. It eventually came to court in January 2009 when magistrates said it should never have been brought. Said Mr Khan's lawyer, Simon Farnsworth: 'The parking ticket clearly wasn't left on the street because it is here in court today. It was produced at the town hall within minutes of being put on the windscreen.' Mr Khan was found not guilty of the littering charge and said: 'I'm sure the people who live in the borough can think of much better ways to spend their money.' And commented Barry Segal of the drivers' pressure group Appeal Now: 'This is an astonishing waste of money and a senseless attack on a man who has made real sacrifices in the defence of this country. It is the sort of mindless act by parking officials that upsets members of the public so much.'

In February it was announced that a team of police community support officers which had cost the tax-payer almost £10m had handed out just fifteen fines since its formation three years before. They issued four fines in 2006, one in 2007 and ten in 2008. That works out at a cost to the tax-payer of more than £650,000 per ticket. Ten of the tickets issued by the Lincolnshire squad were for either having a dirty bicycle light or riding on a pavement. The number of PCSOs in the county had risen from 114 at the start to 159 at the height of its 'power' (although that power does not enable them to make arrests). Lincolnshire has the lowest-funded police force in the country and commented a member of its police authority: 'The tax-payers would be alarmed by the details of the PCSOs' performances.' The tax-payers certainly were. One said: 'The average of five fines a year for the whole of Lincolnshire is diabolical. It either means we are a very trustworthy and law-abiding county or they are not using their powers sufficiently.' The officers' success record also included 192 incidents of confiscating alcohol and thirty-four of confiscating tobacco. Raged one councillor, Chris Underwood-Frost: 'People aren't daft – the public know that this is just policing on the cheap. It's like sending the army to Afghanistan without any guns.' He added that the £10m would have paid for seventy full-time police officers. But senior Lincolnshire officers defended the scheme. Said Assistant Chief Constable Elaine Hill: 'Fines are just one part of the menu, and just as important is the use of inter-personal skills to resolve issues . . .'

One would have thought that car company Vauxhall would have found better ways to spend a Government grant of £8.7m it received in March. But someone high up decided part of the money should be used on a team-building exercise – creating fire engines with Lego and drawing farmyard animals. It was aimed at getting the best teamwork out of employees at the car company's Ellesmere Port plant in Merseyside in preparation for getting a new Astra car off the production lines in September. Said one angry worker: 'It's madness. You've got highly-skilled workers playing kids' games. We're car makers, not toy makers.' The 2,000 factory staff were on a four-day week because of the recession and the grant was crucial to aid its production of the Astra. Commented Tory MP David Davies: 'I can't see how making Lego can train you to build an Astra . . .'

It was no laughing matter when motorist Gary Sanders was pulled over by the police in March 2009 and reprimanded for having a chuckle behind the wheel. It was an over-enthusiastic member of the Liverpool force who stopped company director, 47-year-old Mr Sanders as he exited the Mersey Tunnel. Mr Sanders said he had been laughing at a funny comment a friend had made to him over his hands-free car phone. He was told by the officer that 'Laughing while driving a car can be an offence' and was questioned for thirty-five minutes – not just about the 'offence' but about his ethnic group, distinguishing marks on his body and even what colour his hair was. Mr Sanders suffers from alopecia.

Said Mr Sanders: 'I couldn't believe it when the officer told me I'd been pulled over for laughing. He accused me of throwing my head back in a dangerous way. I was astonished that he could say laughing might be an offence. What is the country coming to?'

Commented Brian Gregory from the Association of British Drivers: 'This is a shocking example of the police harassing innocent motorists simply because they are an easy target.'

That same month poor Penny Batkin was forced to pull over in her car and administer emergency treatment to her 4-year-old disabled son Freddie. Her actions were caught on camera but instead of having sympathy for her plight, Richmond Council upheld a £100 fine. For in her haste to help her little boy who was gasping for breath, 40-year-old Mrs Batkin had parked on the pavement. As she had been en route to a children's hospice near her home in Hampton Wick, South-West London, and because of Freddie's obvious need for resuscitation, Mrs Batkin believed her plight justified her appeal against the fine which was imposed by an over-zealous traffic warden. Her appeal letter was even accompanied by a doctor's supportive note. But none of that initially cut any ice with Richmond Council who quoted a section of the Highway Code relating to parking on the pavement and insisted it was not necessary for her to have done so.

Said Mrs Batkin: 'I hadn't parked. I had stopped to deal with an emergency situation.'

Local charity Richmond Aid said it was stunned by the whole affair. Its chief executive Margaret Gallagher said: 'We are just so appalled that we struggle to find the words. Surely a life and death situation has to constitute sufficient cause to allow this lady to tear up the fine.'

Richmond Council later backed down and cancelled the parking ticket, commenting: 'The appeals officer had not fully appreciated the true sense of urgency. We have now reviewed the matter further and have decided to cancel the penalty charge notice. We apologise for any inconvenience or distress caused to Mrs Batkin.'

It was only a publicity photograph for cycle shop Halfords when it presented bikes to Lancashire Police in June as a contribution to the local community. But PC Tony Gobban refused to pose astride his mountain bike because he had not passed his cycling proficiency test. He explained that his force had a stringent health and safety policy. Luckily, community support officer Emma Nixon who HAS passed her test stepped in to help out with the photo-opportunity. Stated Inspector Nick Emmett: 'Our officers are required to be appropriately trained and assessed prior to using bikes for patrolling in order to comply with insurance and for the safety of themselves and the public.' But commented Councillor Geoff Driver, Conservative group leader on Lancashire County Council: 'The mind boggles when a grown man can't go on a bike for a photograph. When I hear stories like this, I just think what on earth is going on . . . ?' Mr Driver was no doubt even more bemused when later that same year, police officers devised a 93-page, two-volume guide called the Police Cycle Training Doctrine for the Association of Chief Police Officers. The guide offered practical tips such as how to get on and off a bike safely, how to turn, stop and balance, avoid kerbs, to look over the shoulder when at a crossing (actual term was 'rear scan') how NOT to arrest suspects while riding your bike – sorry, while 'engaged with the cycle' – and to wear padded shorts 'for in-saddle comfort'. It was also helpfully suggested that officers might like to consider eating and drinking at some time during their patrol to avoid getting hungry and thirsty and that they should carry out a risk assessment if they wanted to ride their bikes without a helmet when 'undercover'. The Association later back-pedalled over being saddled with a guide that also informed cycling officers how to look left and right at a junction – official term 'deployment at a junction' – and said it would not proceed with the project.

A toddler's swipe at a car with a stick ended with her being perhaps the youngest British citizen ever to be investigated by police on suspicion of vandalism. Wiltshire police were called to the 2-year-old's home in Chippenham in June after the vehicle's owner called them and claimed the child – who could barely walk let alone talk – deliberately damaged his car. It later emerged that the toddler's name and address were held on file after the incident – although they would not be added to the national police database and her DNA was not taken. To be fair, the police had found themselves in the middle of a neighbour's dispute and had visited both parties to defuse the situation. A spokesman for Wiltshire Police said: 'Under the Home Office rules, officers must attend where an allegation has been made, irrespective of the accused person's age. They are obliged to do so and they are also required to record the allegation as a crime.

But if the person is under the age of responsibility they cannot be arrested.' But Michelle Elliott, founder of Kidscape commented: 'You cannot have a child of 2 as a suspect. It is insane. It is stupid. This is the most bizarre thing I have heard of. It makes a mockery of the law.'

It would have been the highlight of the July Lord Mayor's Street Procession – that famous film star car 'Chitty Chitty Bang Bang' proudly making its way along the streets of Norwich in Norfolk. Except our fine four-fendered friend did not have an MoT and was therefore banned by the local police. One way around the ban would have been to put the car on a trailer – but that just did not seem right somehow. Said Helen Selleck, events manager for Norwich City Council: 'Although the road is closed for the annual procession, it is still classed as a public highway and the DVLA is clear all the vehicles involved need to be fully covered.'

The police, of course, stood firm with a spokesman saying: 'We have no problem with the vehicle being securely fastened to a trailer so it can feature in the procession but our priority is the safety of the public and we cannot make exceptions, even for this fun, family occasion.'

There was a similar ban in the Hampshire village of Swanmore that same month when the carnival procession was classified as a 'walking parade' without floats and everyone, from the Carnival Queens to the community fund-raisers all going on foot.

The simple explanation was that the people who kindly provide Swanmore with lorries did not have any spare drivers – thanks to the 2007 EU directive governing lorry drivers' working hours. After looking at all the options, organisers Meon Valley Lions Club realised they needed a host of permits and insurance policies for the 800-yard parade.

Said Lions Club president John Sharpe: 'The more we looked into the details, the more we realised it wasn't worth it. The insurance was going to cost more than £50 per float which was prohibitive.'

* * *

It was pensioner Raymond Smith's pride and joy: a chrome-plated brass model of his old boxer dog pet Colonel which graced the bonnet of whatever car he had for nearly fifty years. Colonel the mascot survived bumps and scrapes, a head-on crash with a tractor in the French Alps, an attempt by a thief in Germany to unscrew him from his pride of place and regular attendance at car rallies all over Europe. But he could not escape the long arm of the law which unleashed the threat of a court case if Colonel did not remove himself from Mr Smith's Fiat Panda. Police in the 86-year-old war veteran's home town of Gillingham in Dorset said that the figure of Colonel was a danger to pedestrians who found themselves rolling over the bonnet in an accident. Mr Smith was threatened with a £50 fine and five penalty points on his licence if he failed to conform following being reported to the police by a killjoy. Mr Smith said: 'It seems ridiculous. Nobody has taken any notice of it for fifty years. It is harmless. I got a call from the police who told me I had a dangerous dog on my car. I thought somebody was having me on. But a traffic officer told me it was illegal as it was a potential danger to pedestrians and I had to get rid of it.' Colonel was relegated to the rear parcel shelf in Mr Smith's car. It was not the same, with Mr Smith confessing: 'I feel rather sad about it. Whenever I drive I am used to seeing him sat out on the bonnet leading the way.' Dorchester traffic police officer, PC Terry Swain explained why Colonel had to go, saying: 'Objects on the bonnets of Mercedes and Rolls Royces are designed to bend or come off in crashes. Fixed, solid objects on bonnets are a safety issue because they can cause increased injury to pedestrians if they were in a collision and rolled over the bonnet.'

Motorists stuck bumper to bumper on the A338 in Bournemouth, Dorset found no solace in the knowledge that the reason for their hour-long delays was also having a slow day . . . For slow-worms are protected under UK and European laws and were being rescued from their natural habitat before £26m of roadworks could take place. Pleas from local traders to put the eight-week slow-worm mission on hold until after Christmas and thus encourage rather than deter motorists to shop in the town, fell on deaf ears. Dorset County Council said the rescue operation had to be done while the reptiles were hibernating. Said Tony Brown, chief executive of the town's Beales department store: 'It's daft they are doing this at this time of the year. The dual carriageway is chock-a-block for miles but the actual stretch they are using is only about 150 yards. They should be doing this in January which is the slowest economic time of the year.' The dual carriageway was reduced to a single lane for nearly 7 miles, a hold-up justified by David Diaz, the council's project manager for the scheme because 'we are governed by legislation as to how we treat these species of animals. Some of them are protected by European legislation as well'. One annoyed driver, self-named on a local internet forum as 'Irate Commuter' wrote: 'If I dressed in a lizard costume, would I get a police escort through the roadworks?' A spokesman for the Amphibian and Reptile Conservation in Bournemouth admitted the situation could be 'pretty irritating' but said that Dorset has the most 'important populations of these species in the country'.

Don't rely on a passing friendly copper to help you change a flat tyre. Well, not if you come under the Metropolitan Police areas anyway. Because they are not allowed to change their own flat tyres. That's why one day in November 2009, two probably rather embarrassed police officers were spotted in their patrol car in Surbiton, South London, waiting for help. It eventually came in the form of VT Critical Services, a private firm contracted by the Met to be on 24-hour call to aid with maintenance of all the Met police's 3,600 vehicles. And that includes changing a tyre. Had the two officers had a go at doing the job themselves, they would have been disciplined for going against 'police procedure'. Commented Peter Smyth, chairman of the Metropolitan Police Federation: 'It isn't logical. If there's a spare wheel in the vehicle and there's a jack, you don't need to be a mechanic to change the wheel . . . that vehicle and those officers are out of commission for an hour or two and that's not the best use of resources. I'd like to see some common sense.' Justifying the contract firm, a spokesman for the Met Police said: 'Police vehicles are maintained to very high standards as they are subject to continual and demanding use 24/7. For these reasons tyres are changed by specialist contractors.'

It was a bitter blow for motorist Michael Mancini when he blew his runny nose while stuck in a traffic queue. For 39-year-old furniture restorer and father of two Mr Mancini ended up with a £60 on-the-spot fine and three penalty points on his driving licence after being accused of not being 'in proper control of his vehicle'. He was, as one might imagine, not a happy man, storming: 'I was just completely gobsmacked . . . I made sure it was safe. The traffic was nose to tail in the high street. We came to a complete stop and I thought that was quite a good time to blow my nose. I stopped the van and put the handbrake on. The traffic moved on and I was waved across by an officer. I still had the tissue in my hand and was stunned when he said I was getting a fixed penalty notice. Surely it would have been more dangerous to drive with a blocked nose?' The incident was on course for an appearance by Mr Mancini at Ayr District Court when he refused to pay the fine and despite a letter from his solicitor Mr Peter Lockhart explaining the circumstances. Commented Mr Lockhart: 'In the letter we sent I said it should have been obvious to the officers what was going on and that it beggars belief a ticket was issued. I also wrote that given the circumstances we cannot see how this case is in the public interest.' The officer involved in the case is no stranger to controversy. Nicknamed PC Shiny Buttons because of his over-enthusiastic approach to his job, Strathclyde policeman Stuart Gray was the man who issued a £50 fixed penalty notice to unemployed Stewart Smith for littering after he accidentally dropped a £10 note in the street as he left a shop (see Keeping Up

Appearances). It was also the same police force who stopped motorist Gary Sanders for laughing in his car (see on page 62).

In January 2010, it took magistrates just five minutes to dismiss a case against 34-year-old Avon and Somerset police officer Duncan Verel who had been accused of knocking a fleeing drug dealer off his bicycle. The court decided that convicted criminal, 23-year-old Somalian national Ibrahim Nur had given evidence 'riddled with inaccuracies and untruths' and that PC Verel was not deserving of being charged with driving without due care and attention – a charge he strongly denied. He said he had not rammed his unmarked police car into Nur's bike even once, let alone the three times Nur claimed, sending him flying into the air, and that the drug dealer had lost his balance trying to get away. PC Verel was on duty on November 28th 2009 when he got a call to assist a colleague trying to apprehend Nur. The ensuing chase ended with Nur falling under the car and being taken to hospital with leg injuries. He underwent skin grafts to his thighs. Collision investigator Sergeant David Loat told the court: 'On the evidence of the CCTV it is unlikely the police vehicle was driven in the manner described by Mr Nur. There is no indication it was driven in a stop-start manner. It is improbable the impact occurred how Mr Nur said, in that he was thrown into the air. There was no evidence of damage on the bike to show this might be the case. His injuries are not consistent with what he has suggested.' Nur's claim that the accident had left him walking on crutches was knocked down when magistrates in Poole, Dorset, were shown footage of him apparently scoring four goals in a soccer match between Somali youths and a police XI after the accident. PC Verel was naturally relieved to at last see an end to the incident which had seen him suspended from normal duties and under a cloud for fourteen months while he waited for the case to come to court. Paul Budd, of the Avon and Somerset Police Federation, criticised the investigation carried out by the Independent Police Complaints Commission that led to the charge. He said: 'This is yet another example of a police officer appearing in court as a result of performing their duty only for the case to be withdrawn or for the officer to be vindicated when the full facts are properly considered. Police officers, from time to time, become the subject of a complaint but many that come to the fore end up with the officer being vindicated or there not being enough evidence.' Mr Budd added that having spoken to PC Verel 'there were some concerns about the validity of the evidence given by the "victim" in this case. It is important that officers have confidence in the IPCC in the same way that the public do. The IPCC investigated the complaint and they passed it on to the CPS who made the decision to take PC Verel to court based on the evidence. But there was evidence available that would have shown that this wasn't a suitable case to come to court, yet he (PC Verel) still found himself in court.' Commented Tory MP David Davies: 'Once again, the law appears to be on the side of the criminal. This case should never have been brought to court.'

It was traumatic enough for part-time courier 30-year-old Sarah McDonald-Lee to see her car being driven away by a thief with her 3-year-old daughter Sophie strapped in the back seat – but Mrs McDonald-Lee's follow-up experience really drove her over the edge. For she had to pay £150 to get her Vauxhall Zafira car back because it had been 'abandoned'. The unhappy incident happened after Mrs McDonald-Lee left the keys in the ignition as she delivered a parcel in January 2010 in Retford, Nottinghamshire. An opportunist car-jacker leapt into the vehicle and drove off at speed. Luckily, after a desperate 999 call the car and little Sophie were found a mile away, both safe and sound. Mrs McDonald-Lee could not thank the police enough for their prompt help and taking the incident seriously enough to have the car towed away for forensic examination. But then she got a letter from the car recovery firm hired by Nottinghamshire Police. Because the vehicle had been 'abandoned' she had to pay £150 to get it back. There was a warning that she could be charged £20 a day storage. Mrs McDonald-Lee at first quite naturally thought there had been some mistake – she was the innocent victim, not the criminal. But when she contacted the police she was told it was 'policy' to charge car-owners for vehicle recovery. Said Mrs McDonald-Lee: 'I feel I've been treated more like a common criminal than the victim of a terrible crime. It is every mother's worst nightmare. I went to hell and back before we found Sophie. The thief actually looked directly in my face as he jumped into the car. I was screaming "No, no – not my baby". He must have heard me, but he tore down the road with smoke pouring from the wheels.' Mrs McDonald-Lee and her 27-year-old fire officer (and former police officer) husband Dan paid up but lodged an official complaint with the Independent Police Complaints Commission. She added: 'Living with the memory of this is bad enough without being punished. If the police want someone to pick up the bill they ought to track down the thief. He's the one who stole the car and dumped it. They should admit that they have made a mistake.' A police spokesman said that the force's policy meant owners had to pay when abandoned vehicles were recovered from the roadside as 'These matters are set down in legislation'.

In March, a specially-trained team terrifyingly wielding more powers than your everyday traffic warden hit the streets controlled by North Lincolnshire Council for a dummy run to catch out motorists who left their engines running (as well as other minor offences such as parking on a double yellow line). Had the team really been up-and-running during that trial fortnight they would have successfully scooped £25,000 in fines for the 500 warning tickets they issued – quite a haul compared to the local Humberside Police issuing 1,081 for the whole of 2009. The team became 'official' on March 1st 2010, with similar teams being introduced throughout the country over the next year. A Government report said that the scheme was mainly aimed at lorry drivers who leave their engines running while loading and unloading. But car drivers were subject to fines too for committing the offence. The idea behind the scheme was to help reduce carbon monoxide emissions and balance climate change. A spokesman for the innovatory North Lincolnshire Council said: 'The council would not target motorists who leave engines running for just a few seconds', adding that fines would only be issued if the public refused to co-operate. At the same time, it did not like 'irresponsible drivers who are not considering the environment'. There were some – as well as motorists of course – who were nearly driven over the edge by the whole thing. Nigel Humphries of the Association of British Drivers said: 'It's just an absolutely ridiculous money-making scam. Engines do not use much fuel when they are idling.'

5

Politically Correct, Laughingly Wrong

It is probably Britain's most popular pastime – and many a father has introduced his son to the pleasures of fishing. But all that looked destined to end when Brussels bureaucrats, determined to protect endangered species and impose fish quotas, were angling to include amateur fishermen in their rules. The reasoning, insisted Joe Borg, commissioner for maritime affairs and fisheries, was that 'Enforcement of catch limits should be the cornerstone of the fisheries policy. The future of sustainable fisheries requires us to replace a system which is inefficient, with one that produces results.' That would mean that not only would boat skippers have to register their boats and stop fishing when they reached their quota, but so too would 1.4m UK sea anglers. Said sea angler Mike Thrussell: 'I'm not the slightest bit surprised that bureaucrats in Brussels are pushing to have sea anglers included in commercial quotas. They have a history of not doing any proper research. They look at the quoted 1.4m UK sea anglers and assume – wrongly as usual – that we're all killing a multitude of fish. It's the recreational sea anglers that have been banging on about the overkill of fish stocks by the commercial fisherman for nearly three decades and nobody listened . . .'

In January, too, Conservative South Cambridgeshire District Council announced plans to spend up to £500,000 building a noise barrier to make life more pleasant for a group of travelling folk who had complained about the nuisance of passing cars and motorists. The fifty-strong group said their lives had been made a misery with constant beeps of abuse, the shouting of obsceni-ties and the flashing of lights as vehicles passed their Blackwell encampment by the A14 near Milton in Cambridgeshire. The camp was opened as a transit site in the 1970s and became an official council-run facility in 1993. It secured a £15,000 grant to improve the entrance to the camp and then felt it necessary to install a noise barrier to protect the residents. Said Sebastian Kindersley, the leader of the LibDem opposition: 'The travellers live between a motorway and a rubbish dump – it must be pretty desperate and something should be done urgently. They are entitled to their privacy.' Added Nick Wright, the councillor responsible for planning: 'It's such a noisy place to live. When you go down there it's almost a job just to have a conversation.' But commented Mark Wallace of the TaxPayers' Alliance: 'Given that the residents of this site are self-declared travellers, it is amazing that they do not simply move on somewhere else if they don't like the fact they are living next to a dual carriageway. There is very little reason why tax-payers should bear a massive bill because of the surroundings people have chosen for them-selves . . .'

Relations between householders and travellers had not had the best start to the year in another Cambridgeshire village, that of Cottenham. The residents had learned to live alongside one of Britain's biggest traveller camps but they were not happy to hear that local officials were spending £8,000 of Lottery cash to teach local children Romany songs – with a view to putting on a show at the end of the year to unite both groups. Pupils from Cottenham Village College and Cottenham, Waterbeach and Willingham primary schools were taught for four half-days each by two musicians from the East Anglian Music Trust. Said Amy Wornald, arts development manager for Fen Edge Community Association: 'The traveller community has been based in Cottenham for generations. We are really keen to revive the songs that arrived here with travellers so they can be shared by the whole community. There has been a lot of tension over the years between the settled and travelling communities and I think it's really important that people share their heritage.' One mother simply said: 'I am sure there are a lot of people around the village who would have appreciated that money for better causes.'

Travellers' tales continued with the announcement that organisers of London's 2012 Olympic Games were spending nearly £2m to requisition a travellers' camp and rehouse the inhabitants. The travelling folk were moved into luxury homes (complete with driveways to accommodate their caravans) on an exclusive gated development. This followed the decision to turn the council-owned site in Hackney Wick, East London, into a handball arena. The London Development Agency was behind the controversial move. It had previously come under fire for spending £3 million building an upmarket camp for seven traveller pitches nearby. Justifying their actions, a spokesman said: 'There were no existing sites to accommodate these families so the new travellers' site was selected in consultation with Hackney Council following an extensive search of the local area.' To be fair, the travellers were being asked to pay £104.66 rent for the three-bedroom homes as well as £9.23 to park their caravan. The question was, of course, would they pay it? Stormed one resident: 'I thought the whole idea of being a traveller was that you lived in a caravan and travelled – not in a bungalow paid for by tax-payers.' There was also the criticism that with so many empty homes in the capital, building new ones for such a cause was unacceptable. By February 2009, the Olympics budget had soared to £9.3billion – four times the original estimate.

And in October, a High Court judge caused outrage by ruling that six traveller families did not act in a 'cynical or ruthless way' when they built an illegal site on green belt land over the Easter holiday weekend. Stormed Keith Parker, who was chairman of Brentwood Borough Council's planning committee when the site was built: 'They never came and asked for advice from the council. They just arrived on site. It's a normal ploy. It's difficult to explain to the general public that their conservatory, their extension or balcony doesn't comply with planning legislation when another group of people can ride roughshod over it.' The travellers were believed to have bought the three-acre site at Blackmore, Essex, from a fellow traveller on April 9th and then the following day, Good Friday, brought along trucks and gone on to lay 1,000 tons of hardcore creating plots for twelve caravans housing seventeen adults and three children. The first the council knew about it was when officers returned to work after the Easter break. They ordered that further work should stop and later refused a planning application on the grounds it was inappropriate green belt development. The travelling families lodged an appeal against the refusal, scheduled to be heard in January 2010. But in October judge Mr Justice Stadlen rejected the council's application to evict the travellers, saying they had acted with the 'best intentions to comply with planning law' and added that they had a good chance of winning planning permission because the hardship of evicting them outweighed the damage to the environment. The travellers themselves admitted they had broken the law but blamed the council for not supplying enough legal sites for them. But said local MP Eric Pickles: 'It just shows how out of touch the judiciary is on these issues. The people of Blackmore will feel the law has let them down and they are right. It shows that use of force and direct action has trodden the rights of the people of Blackmore into the dust. The law needs to be changed.'

She was the church choir member and arts and crafts teacher who was a pillar of the community in Kenton, near Exeter, Devon until she caught teenage vandals running amok in the flower beds she had planted on the village green. Now 63-year-old Alma Harding has a criminal record. For when she spotted the three teenagers kicking a ball among the flowers she called to them to stop, only to be greeted with the response of abuse and swearing. Mrs Harding became fearful of attack and lashed out with the copy of a church minutes' meeting she had in her hand. One 13-year-old boy was caught on the cheek. Mrs Harding was then charged with battery and convicted at Newton Abbot Magistrates Court. Defending Mrs Harding, James Taghdissian said that she had just been trying to prevent the green being vandalised and that because she is small, she felt intimidated by being surrounded by three teenage boys. There was also a history of vandalism in the village with windows, plants and railings having been damaged.

Mrs Harding admitted hitting the boy with the paper but denied slapping him with her hand. But she was found guilty as they said her actions had not been in self-defence. Mrs Harding was given an absolute discharge, meaning she left court unpunished, but still with a criminal record.

Magistrates chairman Catherine French said: 'She is clearly committed to the community where she lives. We find that words were exchanged and the boys laughed while standing in front of her. She did strike him with the paper. But her feelings were exasperated by acts of vandalism. We find she did not act in self-defence.' The court did not award compensation to the victim because there was 'no distress or injury'. After the hearing Mrs Harding, who spent £2,270 on legal costs, said she did what anyone would have done. 'You can't even tell kids off without being arrested. Their parents should be keeping them under control.'

And Mr Taghdissian said the court's decision sent out the 'wrong message to anyone taking a stand' and added: 'Mrs Harding did not accept an earlier caution she was offered because she does not accept she did anything wrong. You can see the effect it has had on her already. She has lost her good name. Why is the Crown Prosecution wasting time and money on this case? The message this sends out to young people in our society is that they can conduct themselves in this way knowing that anyone who takes a stand will end up in the dock.'

Someone else who had a brush with the law while trying to uphold it was 49-year-old courier driver Roland Digby who tried to make a citizen's arrest when his house was pelted with apples by a gang of youths. Father of three Mr Digby ended up facing court having been charged with common assault after allegedly placing his hand on the shoulder of a 16-year-old trying to restrain him. There was some swearing from the aggrieved teenager, a scuffle and a fray involving around fifteen other teenagers. When Mr Digby finally broke free he complained to two passing policemen who told him to go home and wait for official police response. There wasn't one that night on September 3rd, but five days later Mr Digby was arrested at his home in Royston, Hertfordshire after he refused to accept a caution. Mr Digby spent several hours in a cell, endured a court appearance and lost three days of work before the Crown Prosecution Service decided there was no realistic prospect of a prosecution. Its chief prosecutor for Hertfordshire, David Robinson said: 'There was insufficient evidence to prove that Mr Digby used unreasonable and excessive force or that he was acting unreasonably. Reasonable force can be used in self-defence of property, prevention of crime or when making lawful arrest.' Mr Digby, who had been forced to take matters into his own hands after three consecutive nights of harassment from the young gang, accused Hertfordshire Police of 'hounding me when they could have been catching real criminals' adding: 'Common sense seems to have prevailed. It's just a shame they had to put myself and my family through this first. It all comes down to the fact police did not come and get both sides of the story before they charged me.' On the night in question Mr Digby and his wife had made four 999 calls before Mr Digby decided to tackle the youths himself. He added: 'It was madness they even charged me and clearly madness they took me to court. This has been hanging over me for almost a month – it's been terrifying.'

There was another case of the abuse of 'flower power' that June after it was reported that former care worker Jane Clift, 43, reported a drunk she saw trampling plants in Sheffield Road Rest Gardens, Slough, Bucks, and had ended up with a four-year legal battle to clear her name. The trouble had started way back in August 2005 when Mrs Clift called police to the scene but the drunk had left by the time they arrived. They advised her to contact Slough Council which was running a campaign to persuade local people to report anti-social behaviour. Mrs Clift's frustration at getting no action there saw her taking her complaint to a more senior level – a level in the shape of one Fozia Rashid who claimed Mrs Clift was 'very difficult' and had been rude to her. A few months later, Mrs Clift received a letter from the council saying she had been put on the register of potentially violent persons. She had no previous criminal record but was now forced to abandon her plans to become a foster parent after her details were circulated to a large range of public and private bodies including doctors, dentists, opticians, libraries, family planning clinics, schools and nurseries. The staff at all were advised not to see Mrs Clift on their own. It was no wonder Mrs Clift decided to leave the town where she had lived for ten years. She said: 'My whole life was destroyed. It was impossible to function normally in the town. All it takes is one council buffoon to take a dislike to you and he or she can put you on this register.' The High Court ordered Slough Council to pay Mrs Clift £12,000 in libel damages after the case which cost tax-payers around £500,000 in legal fees – to be paid for by Slough Council as ordered by Mr Justice Tugendhal. Mrs Clift's counsel, Hugh Tomlinson said an angry letter from her to the council had been misinterpreted and the decision to put her name on such a register was a bid for no-one to take her seriously because she was a 'thorn in their side'. Commented Simon Davies, from human rights watchdog Privacy International: 'It is the sort of behaviour that we would have condemned if it came from China or Russia. Our councils seem to be out of control.' A spokesman for Slough Council said: 'The jury found that what we recorded about Mrs Clift was not true, but they were not prepared to find we acted in bad faith. We will reflect carefully on how we need to respond.'

* * *

Another pillar of the community, popular head teacher Julia Robinson resigned in January after parents objected to her replacing separate assemblies for Muslim pupils with a single gathering for all faiths. Chairman of the school governors, Sarah Browton, also resigned in support. Mrs Robinson had been accused of racism, was laid off from working at the school for nearly a year and finally left following protests against her by a small number of parents. Yet she had sought advice from education chiefs about her plan for her school, Meersbrook Bank Community Primary in Sheffield, where most of the pupils are white Christians – with about thirty-five Muslim children. Mrs Robinson believed her change would promote 'inclusiveness' in the multi-cultural school. It was claimed that the problems began when hymns were introduced to the single assemblies, an inclusion objected to by the Muslims who said they wanted a non-secular assembly. 'We felt we were being marginalised,' said one. 'We didn't put any pressure on her. We want continuity at the school. It was her decision to leave.' Commented one parent: 'Mrs Robinson was hounded out. Very few people objected to the changes. But it seems people are scared of Muslims.'

Meanwhile, a foster mother was struck off the register for allowing a Muslim girl in her care to convert to Christianity. The woman – whose identity was not disclosed for legal reasons – had looked after more than eighty children, claimed to have put no pressure on the teenage girl and stated that social workers had raised no objections to her own beliefs. She said: 'I did initially try to discourage her (the girl). I offered her alternatives. I offered to find places for her to practise her own religion. I offered to take her to friends and family. But she said to me from the word go "I am interested and I want to come."' But officials did object to the girl being baptised, saying the foster mother had failed in her duty to preserve the girl's religion and should have tried to stop the baptism. They also said the girl should stay away from church for six months. The woman launched a legal battle over her case, financially backed by the Christian Institute, whose reasoning was: 'All people should be free to change or modify their religious beliefs . . . I cannot imagine that an atheist foster carer would be struck off if a Christian child in her care stopped believing in God. This is the sort of double standard which Christians are facing in modern Britain.'

The trademark of singer Al Jolson was his blacked-up face. So it made sense that when telling his story such detail was kept in for an accurate portrayal. But Michael Harrison, producer of the musical *Jolson & Co* did not agree. He said: 'Blacking-up is historically correct, but in this day and age we are not out to offend anyone. There is a reference to blacking-up in the script, but we didn't feel it was necessary to include it within the show.'

And so it was that actor Allan Stewart played the part of a blacked-up singer without the blacking when he took to the stage in Edinburgh in February 2009. Mr Stewart was a bit miffed about the make-up ban. He said: 'I personally believe it should be in there, but even the slightest sign of negativity could be bad for the show.' The actor had played Jolson twelve years earlier in London and said that although there were initially a few protesters outside the theatre, they had been won over when they actually saw the show.

Actors' union Equity said that although it was normally opposed to actors blacking-up, this was one instance when it was deemed acceptable 'because it is about a white artist who blacked-up'. And the Campaign Against Political Correctness agreed, with spokesman Richard Cook saying: 'It's a case of producers being oversensitive. Most people who attend an Al Jolson tribute will know his background but the show they are going to see will be incomplete in terms of its historical accuracy.'

In February too, librarians were told to move the Muslim 'bible' the Koran, to a top shelf because followers of Islam said it should be put above commonplace things. In an attempt to bring equality to all religions, the librarians then decided the Bible should go on the top shelf too – only to cause upset to Christians who felt it should be within their reach. It all started when the Museums, Libraries and Archives Council reported that Muslims in Leicester had moved copies of the Koran to the top shelves of libraries because the word of God was so important. The city's librarians then consulted the Federation of Muslim Organisations and were advised that all religious texts should be kept on the top shelf. Their guiding advice was: 'This means that no offence is caused as the scriptures of all the major faiths are given respect in this way, but none is higher than the other.' Critics said this stance saw religious works being revered rather than readily available to read. Said Robert Whelan of the Civitas group: 'Libraries and museums are not places of worship. They should not be run in accordance with particular religious beliefs.' Added Simon Chivers of the Christian Institute: 'I hope there will be a rethink. I understand that Muslims revere their own text, but in public libraries there should not be a policy of putting religious texts out of reach.'

In March 2009, postmaster Deva Kumarasiri was transferred for asking customers to speak English. He caused a storm of controversy when he banned non-English-speaking customers from his sub-post office in Sneinton Boulevard, Carlton, Nottingham. Sri Lankan-born Mr Kumarasiri said that he believed immigrants should learn to speak the language of the country in which they are now residing. But his stance upset some of the local Muslim community and angered his boss, Rizwan Raja who owns the shop in which the post office is sited. Mr Raja said: 'We have been trying to build up the business. It does not matter about race or language. If we can help people, we will.'

Mr Kumarasiri who has been in Britain for eighteen years was transferred to a secret post office location following a petition signed by Muslims to oust him and amidst fear of reprisals.

But he was adamant about his belief, saying: 'I'm not backing down. It's only a few people who have forced me out. It's not the people out there. They support me.

'I didn't impose a complete ban. I told people to learn some English or come back with an interpreter. They come back now with the right attitude.'

Mr Kumarasiri was inundated with cards and messages of support but lost his job as local councillor for the Liberal Democrats. But he stood his ground and said: 'If these people are coming into our country they should practise our language and culture. As far as I am concerned, if you can't be British, you should go home. I don't expect everyone to agree with me. But this proves that there are elements out there who have no intention of ever being integrated.' Shortly afterwards, Mr Kumarasiri was sacked.

In March, Paul and Deborah Rees were awarded a £4,550 Government grant to help set themselves up in business. They must have seen it coming. For Deborah, 37, and Paul, 40, received the money through a Department for Work and Pensions job creation scheme to support their careers as clair-voyants at their Accolade Academy of Psychic and Mediumistic Studies. The academy trains people to contact 'the other side'. The couple, who run £65 medium workshops from their home in Bridgend, South Wales, admitted that despite their psychic powers the grant still came as a surprise. Said Paul, who with his wife, had to prove a psychic talent before receiving the money: 'People who feel their tax money has been wasted should remember that if they'd lost a child they would go to a medium to get peace that their loved one has passed safely and is in a better place.' The TaxPayers' Alliance, always ready to defend the way our money is spent, commented that the last thing it should go on is 'this kind of hocus pocus . . . At a time when people who are alive are losing their jobs, it's absurd that money is being spent to contact the other side.'

It's been sung for centuries and stirs the heart. But as far as the BBC was concerned, the National Anthem just did not sum up the country well enough and lacked a modern twist. That is why it came up with its own anthem which included the words: 'I am England – England is inside of me. I am England – England is what I want Her to be . . .' The BBC teamed up with the Arts Council England to create its alternative 'God Save the Queen' which was included in a production called *The Full English*. The song was the work of folk musician Sam Dunkley and was intended to 'reflect English customs, ideas and creativity in contemporary times'.

A glimpse of just two lines of the song prompted Conservative MP Ann Widdecombe to comment: 'As far as I am concerned, the National Anthem should stay exactly as it is, which is fine. Secondly, those lines are so banal that even an 11-year-old would disown them. I am perfectly happy to be British and perfectly happy with the National Anthem as it is. I certainly don't aspire to rewrite anything.'

The politically correct ditty was defended by Janet Robertson, creative director of *The Full English*, who said: 'It was decided that music is the single greatest unifying force, something to which everyone – regardless of race, creed or class – can respond. The group has been talking to a wide range of people to find out what, for them, typifies England and trying to incorporate this into the anthem. The result aims to be a song for everyone, a celebratory moment that reveals what people think is good about England.' The song also contained a reference to onion bhajis as well as the lines 'Swing low sweet chariot, God Save the Queen.' The song was performed by schoolchildren on St George's Day and according to Mr Dunkley: 'It went brilliantly and there was a huge energy from the children. We talked about what England means to them, to young people in the modern day and that's what came out of it. Simple things which appealed to children.'

In March, Oxfordshire's social services decided that £20,000 should be spent on ensuring their care homes are 'gay-friendly'. The major plan included re-arranging furniture in the homes so that gay couples could have a cuddle.

The traditional Easter bonnet parade was cancelled at Meersbrook Bank Primary School in Sheffield. No official reason was given, but parents suspected it was linked to previous outrage from the thirty-five Muslim pupils who had complained when the former head teacher had tried to encourage all the school's 240 children to attend a multi-faith assembly. Now Easter was just too Christian. Even one Muslim mother was baffled, saying 'if that's the reason then it's daft and nit-picking. Children go to school to learn and making Easter bonnets is fun. I don't see the problem. If it's got some religious connection, so what?' And commented Mike Judge of the Christian Institute: 'How can it be offensive to celebrate a Christian festival in a Christian country? So often these things are done by somebody who feels they should be offended on somebody else's behalf. In reality, other religious groups are as baffled as the rest of us by this politically correct nonsense.'

All the chairman of the school governors, Mr Rob Stephens, would say is that the ban on bonnets was a 'staff decision because there were so many things going on at once'.

It was also in April that year, that a school caused major outrage by giving its pupils lessons in bad language to 'dispel the myths of swear-words'. Words that would make parents – and all other respectable people – wince were written on boards and had their meanings explained in health education lessons to 11 and 12-year-olds (who were also asked to shout out slang words for sex and certain parts of the body). One teacher refused to take part in the lessons at St Laurence School in Bradford on Avon, Wiltshire. Said one angry parent: 'This is a total disgrace. We send our children to school to gain an education, not qualifications in swear-words. Most of the children in that class had no idea what these words meant and have now been forced to grow up faster than their parents would like.'

Deputy head teacher Mr Richard Clutterbuck later apologised for the swearing but added: 'Part of the programme is to ensure students use the correct terms when referring to the biological aspects of the programme and to dispel any use of slang terms. With hindsight, the delivery of this particular lesson should not have focused upon the slang terms and I must apologise for any distress caused.' According to a spokesman for Wiltshire county council, Government guidelines said sex education lessons should allow children to learn, in 'age-appropriate ways' throughout their school career about how they are changing physically and emotionally. 'Part of this is exploring the correct and incorrect language to describe sex and parts of the body.'

That same month, officials were accused of playing fast and loose with a fast-food shop. Jamaican café The Bamboo Joint in Leytonstone, East London, became the first takeaway in the country to be given a 'closure order' under guidelines banning the sale of fast food near educational establishments. Its owners were given three days to shut up shop and end their serving of jerk chicken 400 metres away from a secondary school, 200 metres away from a primary school and 100 metres from a public park. To ensure The Bamboo Joint discontinued its wicked trade, eight police officers, some wearing anti-stab vests, joined three employees of Waltham Forest Council standing on the café doorstep. It was all a bitter blow for one of the owners, Maureen Farrell who had only opened up for business six weeks before. She said the council was acting 'completely over the top' and that she felt victimised because the busy high street was home to many takeaways, fish and chip shops and burger bars. No doubt feeling the 'no jerk' rules were drawn up by, well, jerks, Ms Farrell added: 'It's ridiculous. They just arrived here this morning and told us they were shutting us down. It looks like we are terrorists or something. All we are doing is selling good food and it's not greasy stuff. And we hardly have any schoolchildren in here at all.' The bylaw – intended to cut down child obesity by restricting the number of takeaways in the borough's town centres – was introduced by Waltham Forest in March and applied only to those takeaways yet to receive planning permission. But it was being watched carefully by other authorities. Said Council leader Clyde Loakes: 'This fast-food outlet has not got planning permission and has absolutely no chance of getting it because of its proximity to a park and a school, so we are closing it down. A lot of fast-food outlets do their business with schoolchildren in competition with the healthy schools agenda. We have a responsibility to look beyond the next year or two to the health of our children and young people.'

In June it was reported that police were stopping and searching innocent white people under anti-terror laws to avoid being accused of being racially prejudiced against Asians. Lord Carlile QC, the Government's independent reviewer of anti-terror laws said it was 'totally wrong' and 'gross invasion' as well as 'almost certainly unlawful'. He added: 'I can well understand the concerns of the police that they should be free from allegations of prejudice but it is not a good use of precious resources if they waste them on self-evidently unmerited searches. It is also an invasion of civil liberties of the person who has been stopped simply to "balance" the statistics. If, for example, fifty blonde women are stopped who fall nowhere near any intelligence-led terrorism profile, it's a gross invasion of the civil liberties of those fifty blonde women . . .'

Patients with a permanent roof over their head were left feeling sick when it was announced in June that gypsies and travellers should be given priority in NHS hospitals and doctors' surgeries. The order came from the NHS Primary Care Commissioning, an advisory service for local health trusts, in its Primary Care Service Framework. The body decreed that gypsies will be 'fast-tracked' for doctors, nurses and even some dentist appointments above all other patients. GPs were also told to see any travelling folk who walk in without an appointment, even if all their slots were full for the day. Could it get even worse for long-suffering people who choose to have a permanent home? Well, yes. The gypsy community will also be given longer consultation times than other patients – twenty minutes compared to the usual five or ten – and can be accompanied by their relatives. An extract from the Primary Care Service Framework stated: 'It is important that Gypsies and Travellers are, wherever possible, fast-tracked into primary care services – recognising the fact that they may be forced to move on, and thereby be denied access . . . Walk-in appointments: practices should adopt a policy of not turning away any Gypsy/Traveller who attends without an agreed appointment, even if all appointments for that day are full . . .' It was further decided that staff should be given 'mandatory cultural awareness' training so they can understand what it is like being a traveller or gypsy. But, commented Tory health spokesman Andrew Lansley: 'No-one should get priority in the NHS apart from our Armed Forces to whom we owe a special debt of gratitude. Decisions about who should be treated first should be based on a patient's medical needs, not their ethnic group.' Added Mark Wallace from the TaxPayers Alliance: 'This kind of special treatment is totally uncalled-for and utterly unjustified. The NHS is meant to treat people equally no matter who they are or whatever their race. The only priority should be how ill someone is, not their politically correct concerns.' The new guidelines – which covered groups such as bargees, circus and fairground showmen as well as gypsies and travellers – were justified by the Department of Health who said: 'The Framework suggests fast-tracking for two reasons. First, as a matter of urgency, inroads need to be made into the health problems of gypsies and travellers. Second, if mobile community members are not seen quickly, the opportunity could be lost as they move on or are moved on. This should not be to the detriment of service provision to the settled community.'

Shortly afterwards, it was announced that gypsy and traveller children should be given priority to popular state schools even though there may be a long waiting list of 'resident' children; that they could be registered at two schools at once so that a place could be kept open for them at one while they attend another and that schools should think very carefully about expelling a traveller child. Said a spokesman for the Department for Children, Schools and Families: 'The vast majority of children get a place at their first choice school, but it is absolutely right that disadvantaged groups can get back on track with their education quickly when they move to a new area. Everyone, regardless of background, should have fair and equal access to a place of their choice.' Mr Mark Wallace of the TaxPayers' Alliance said: 'It is absolutely wrong to distribute any public service preferentially on the basis of race. These are public services that tax-payers fund and we should all have to abide by the rules. This kind of positive discrimination is harmful and deeply unfair.' Or, as one aggrieved parent put it: 'I had to wait eighteen months for a place at the school for my child. Now someone can come in and just go to the school. Is that fair?'

In July, pagan police officers persuaded the Home Office to let them set up a support group. The Pagan Police Association is aimed at helping officers who cast spells and join late-night rituals reconcile their beliefs with their police work. Main man behind the group was PC Andy Pardy of Hertfordshire police. An officer for seven years, he is also a heathen who worships Norse gods including Thor and one-eyed Odin. Said PC Pardy: 'A lot of people think it is about dancing naked around a fire but the rituals are not like that. It involves chanting, music, meditation and reading passages. For pagans, these have the same power as prayer does for Christians.' The pagan officers were to be allowed to take off pagan holidays, such as Halloween, from work though this had to be included in their annual leave. The Home Office said that while it was not funding the Pagan Police Association, 'The Government wants a police service that reflects the diverse communities it serves.'

What's in a word? Well, as we have already learned, nowadays it can be quite a lot. And that is why the word 'blacklisting' was banned from use by staff who work for the Citizens Advice Centres. In August the service decreed that the word was offensive and 'fosters stereotypes' and should therefore be changed to 'blocklisting'. Critics said the new rules were daft and simply meant 'political correctness going over the top'. Email references to junk mail should now be accompanied by the word 'blocklisted' instead of 'blacklisted'. Commented a former volunteer within the service (who 'resigned' from his local branch because of this silliness): 'This is the most ridiculous thing I've ever seen.'

Spotted Dick pudding (preferably with custard) has been one of Britain's best-loved comfort foods for years. Ok, so its name might sometimes give rise to childish sniggers for being 'rude' but obviously it refers to the raisins which 'stud' the lovely dough. But in September Flintshire council in North Wales renamed the pud Spotted Richard because it sounded, well, nicer when requested in its town hall menu. But stormed one affronted councillor, Klaus Armstrong Braun: 'I couldn't believe it. It seemed ludicrous. Spotted Dick is part of our heritage. It just seemed political correctness gone mad. There was a sign in the dining room for things like rice pudding and then this Spotted Richard. I had to ask what it was. Whoever has changed it needs to be told they are being silly.' But a spokesman for the council said the change of name came about because of cheeky jokes from diners, adding: 'The correct title for this dish is "Spotted Dick". However, because of several immature comments from a few customers, catering staff have renamed the dish "Spotted Richard" or "Sultana Sponge". This was not a policy decision – staff simply acted as they thought best to put an end to unwelcome and childish comments, albeit from a very small number of customers.'

Shooting games in the playground may not be politically correct – but the last people to know that are the little boys who play them. And that was how 9-year-old Steven Cheek found himself in trouble in September. Having learned about World War II at

Purford Green Junior School in Harlow, Essex, Steven pointed his fingers into a gun at a classmate and said: 'We've got to shoot the German army.' Shortly afterwards Steven was called to see the deputy head accused of being racist because the little boy 'victim' he involved in his game was Polish. Steven had to stand in front of his class and make a public apology and his mother Jane Hennessy was summoned to the school. She was told that her son's behaviour would be a matter of permanent record. Said head teacher Viv Perri: 'When a pupil uses inappropriate language or terms that could be offensive, we have a responsibility to explain to them why their behaviour is wrong. The incident in question involved a short conversation with a pupil to explain the inappropriate nature of his comments and then a meeting with a parent to explain the context.' But explained Miss Hennessy: 'Steven is not a racist. He's only 9 years old and he didn't single out the Polish boy who is one of his good friends. He didn't understand what he had done wrong. He was just playing a game like kids always do. He came home after being told off and said "Mum, what's racism . . . ?"' Commented Nick Seaton of the Campaign for Real Education: 'It's a shame that teachers these days all too often fail to crack down on real problems like bullying but overreact to a child with a healthy imagination.'

It was announced in October that teenage asylum-seekers were being given our money to, er, teach them about our money . . . The weekly £25 pocket money was handed out to youths between 16 and 18 every Friday night by Kent County Council who justified the handouts (amounting to over £50,000 a year) by saying: 'Kent County Council is a gateway authority in Europe. This means we have a high number of asylum-seeking young people in our care who enter the country alone, without their parents or other carers . . . We help newly-arrived asylum-seeking young people to live safely and responsibly in the community. This means, for example, that they are given money so they can learn to use our currency to budget, to shop for food and then to cook safely . . .' It further added of the 900 teenagers either living in foster care or children's homes, that 'the law sets out that they must be treated the same as any other child in the country who is in care and we act as their parent'. Around forty young asylum-seekers are housed by the council in a special reception centre. Commented one irate local resident: 'They get £25 handed to them in a brown envelope while everyone else is fighting to stay afloat. It's a disgrace. They can't wait to get their cash and go out and spend it on things such as cigarettes. If that's learning to use our currency then they're getting very good at it.'

Oh, those days when a certain generation were reassured when TV policeman Dixon of Dock Green bid us 'Evening all . . .' Sadly the current generation will have to do without that friendly phrase. For in October 2009, it was decreed as not just ambiguous but offensive for ethnic groups. New guidelines from Warwickshire police stated that the expression could no longer be used. A spokesman for the force said: 'Terms such as "afternoon" and "evening" are somewhat subjective in meaning and can vary according to a person's culture or nationality. In many cultures, the term evening is linked to the time of the day when people have their main meal of the day. The point is there is an element of subjectivity leading to a variation between cultures that we need to be aware of – taking steps as far as possible to ensure our communication is effective in serving the public.' The new guide also warned against using the words 'businessman', 'housewife', and 'child' (substituting the word 'young person' as all could have 'negative connotations'). But it wasn't just Warwickshire police who had to abide by the new 'law'. The guidelines were also introduced to police forces and fire services throughout the country. The 52-page guide stated that such phrases could have 'connotations of inexperience, impetuosity, and unreliability or even dishonesty'. One woman, Marie Clair, spokesman for the Plain English group, had a few words of her own to say on the matter: 'I have never heard of anyone being confused as to what part of the day it is. When the police need absolute accuracy over when something happened, then I am sure they use the exact time. There comes a point when common sense must prevail.'

When 70-year-old Tony Prior wanted to be helpful and take his housebound neighbour's rubbish to the recycling centre, he was rewarded with an accusation of breaking the law. For he was stopped by staff at the centre in Chard, Somerset, and told he was carrying 'third-party waste' and would have to become a registered carrier. A naturally annoyed Mr Prior said: 'I am outraged. I was just doing a good deed for the day.' A spokesman for Somerset Waste Partnership refused to let their rules be rubbished, however, saying: 'If people knowingly take other people's rubbish to recycling centres they are breaking the law. The only way out of this is for the good Samaritan (that's Mr Prior!) to register with the Environment Agency as a registered carrier. This applies throughout the country.'

In November 2009, a Government-funded report stated that all secondary schools should have a 'gypsy teacher', someone who would mix with travellers, understand their culture, organise days to celebrate great days in the gypsy calendar and above all, give their undivided attention to travelling children. Measures for this included no stringent homework deadlines and the teachers giving out their mobile phone numbers to be on call outside of school hours (a slightly better service than the one given to non-gypsy children, we could say). The idea was mooted after the realisation that travelling children do not attend school regularly and that the majority are unlikely to succeed in exams. The study was compiled for the Government's Department for Children, Schools and Families by the national Foundation for Educational Research, together with the Inner London Traveller Education Consortium. Critics said that with so many 'ordinary' pupils leaving school unable to read or write, funds would be better spent 'on teachers and books to benefit all pupils regardless of social background'.

*   *   *

Throughout history, young lads have been called 'youths' (and the term was good enough for Shakespeare) but in November 2009 an order came from a 'code of practice' issued by the Ministry of Justice and the Department for Children, Schools and Families that lads who have broken the law should be called 'young persons' and not 'youths' as this could offend them. The order noted: 'A number of responses suggested the term "youth" had negative connotations and should be replaced by "young person". Therefore, throughout the code (with the exception of the term "Youth Conditional Caution") "youth" has been replaced.' More than 100 mentions of the 'offensive' word had to be deleted in one document alone – rather embarrassingly in the very code of practice which was issued ordering 'youth' NOT to be used . . .

What is wrong with Christmas? Well, nothing, most of us would agree. But British Transport Police made it a virtual criminal offence to use the word. They dropped the word 'Christmas' from a national poster displayed at railway and underground stations publicising the fact they would still be very much on duty during the season of goodwill and replaced it with the word 'Holiday'. That meant their attempt at a play on words 'Christmas Presence' (presents, get it?) became Holiday Presence which didn't really have the same ring about it. There was a very lengthy explanation from a Transport Police spokesman who said not only was the poster aimed at alerting the public to the fact extra officers were on duty to cope with the traditional rise of assaults on transport staff over the Christmas and New Year period and informing them the penalties were severe but that the strange wording was 'non-denominational so that it applies to everyone and so that people who don't buy into Christmas don't feel excluded'. He added: 'I can see there can be a debate around it but it is a matter of opinion and I am not going to comment. As far as we are concerned, the more publicity we get for the campaign, the better.' The decision to change the wording was made by the Transport Police's marketing manager Alison Lock who was unable to comment as she was away for 'Holiday'. There were many critics of the posters. One, Nick Baines, the Church of England Bishop of Croydon said: 'It is bonkers. To replace the word "Christmas" with "Holiday" not only makes nonsense of the phrase and the sentiment, it also shows that the advertisers have lost the plot.' Added former Tory Minister Ann Widdecombe: 'It's astounding. The person who made this decision must be living on a different planet from everyone else – one where Christmas doesn't exist.' None of this should surprise us. That same month the Tayside city of Dundee promoted its Christmas celebrations as the Winter Night Light festival for politically correct reasons to involve all religions, and the Conservative Party produced Christmas cards wishing everyone 'Season's greetings' and without the word 'Christmas' in case it caused offence – which even its leader, David Cameron said was 'insulting tosh'. New cards were then created bearing the jollier words 'Merry Christmas'.

Little girls and boys alike have enjoyed the antics of the Rev W V Awdry's creation, Thomas the Tank Engine, for many, many years. But then in December 2009, Professor Shauna Wilton put a sexism dampener on the little steam engine and all his friends. For she studied twenty-three video episodes of Thomas and then declared that there were not enough female engines and those there were, tended to be bossy or have 'secondary' roles. Not only that, but the world of Thomas was blighted by a 'conservative political ideology' in which the engines were punished for showing initiative or attempting to better them-selves, and a class divide with Thomas and his friends at the bottom of the social ladder and with their 'Fat Controller' (you have to be a Thomas fan to understand all this) Sir Topham Hatt at the top. In short, Ms Wilton's 3-year-old daughter loved Thomas, but her academic mum did not. The Canadian professor said: 'We tend to think of children's TV shows as neutral and safe, but they still carry messages. Eventually these children will attain full political citizenship, and the opinions and world outlook they develop now, partially influenced by shows like Thomas, are part of that process.' The angst-ridden academic's ideas were criticised by the Campaign Against Political Correctness with spokesman Laura Midgley saying: 'I cannot believe anyone has the time and energy to do such a study. I'm surprised she hasn't singled out the Fat Controller as an example of fattism too. Children should just be left to enjoy the innocent fun of Thomas without the politically correct brigade stoking the fires and ruining their enjoyment.'

Listening to a rock band called 'The Killers' cost mechanic 41-year-old Chris Cureton a £30 fine. For Mr Cureton was told the music coming from the radio in his Vauxhall Astra was too loud, constituting anti-social behaviour. He said: 'I'm not some boy racer with a big sound system fitted in my boot. I'm a dad who was driving home from work listening to some music at what I thought was an acceptable level on my standard factory-fitted car radio. I didn't even know you could get a ticket for playing your radio too loud.' Mr Cureton, from Seacombe, Merseyside appealed against the fine 'on principle' and added: 'If there is a legal level of noise that I exceeded I will willingly pay my fine. When the only evidence is the opinion of a police officer, however, I feel by paying it I could be setting a precedent for laws to be made up as and when it suits the police. I'm still totally baffled and feel like this whole situation is unfair and unjust.'

In December, it was announced that projects in an £800 million, seven-year EU programme Youth in Action to help people 'feel European' included basket-weaving and slapstick acting work-shops. The projects are aimed at those aged 13 to 30 and because the British Government provides 10 per cent of the EU's central budget, a lot of the money is likely to come from tax-payers. And sadly, only a handful of projects benefited young people in Britain – with those such as a coffee house in Finland offering 'everyone the chance to have a sleep for free' and a meeting in Macedonia called Stories and Legends, exploring storytelling. The programme was developed by the European Commission and means that arts and cultural groups can apply for funding after putting forward ideas to the organisation responsible for administering the cash in their home country – in the UK, that is the British Council, from which a spokesman said: 'Projects such as volunteering with homeless charities in Europe give thousands of 13 to 30-year-olds opportunities they would not otherwise get.' And an EC spokesman added: 'I don't see anything wrong with basket-weaving or music-making if it encourages young people to meet other Europeans and learn a new skill from another part of Europe.' None of which impressed campaign group the TaxPayers' Alliance who argued: 'UK tax-payers have a right to know if money is being spent wisely or wasted on frivolity. Given the bizarre projects, it's clearly the latter. But it's worse than just a case of money being squandered. It also shows the lengths to which the EU is seeking to supplant young people's own national identities with a meaningless European identity.'

When model and TV presenter Myleene Klass realised there were intruders in the back garden of her home in Potters Bar, Hertfordshire, one night in January 2010, she called the police straight away. Ms Klass was naturally anxious, particularly as she was alone in the house with her 2-year-old daughter as her fiancé was away at the time. She was further scared when the two youths peered at her through a window and so grabbed a knife from her kitchen and waved it at them. They ran off, leaving tell-tale footprints in the snow behind them.

But far from attempting to track down the villains, the police, upon arrival, warned Ms Klass that she should not have used a knife to warn them off because carrying an offensive weapon, even in her own home, was illegal. Her agent said that Ms Klass had been utterly terrified by the intruders and 'aghast' at the police warning she had received. He said: 'All she did was scream loudly and wave the knife to try and frighten them off. She is not looking to be a vigilante and has the utmost respect for the law, but when the police explained to her that even if you're at home alone and you have an intruder, you are not allowed to protect yourself, she was bemused.' A spokesman for Hertfordshire police said no reference was made in an incident report about a weapon and that it was being treated as trespass with words of advice given 'to ensure suspicious behaviour is reported immediately'.

A month before, the Conservative party pledged it would make it more difficult for people who tackle burglars to be prosecuted. Shadow Home Secretary Chris Grayling spoke out after another householder, 53-year-old businessman Munir Hussain was jailed for thirty months for beating a man who tied up his family at home. Before the sentencing at Reading Crown Court, judge John Reddihough said Mr Hussain had showed great courage in defending his wife and three children from attack and that his family had been subjected to a 'serious and wicked offence' but that Mr Hussain had carried out a 'dreadful, violent attack' on one of the burglars, Walid Salem, as he lay defenceless on the ground.

Mr Hussain, chairman of the Asian Business Council, and his family had returned to their home in High Wycombe, Buckinghamshire to find three intruders wearing balaclavas. Mr Hussain was told he would be killed, his family's hands were tied behind their backs and they were forced to crawl from room to room. Mr Hussain's wife Shaheen told the court: 'They were hitting my husband. When I asked them to stop, they started hitting him again. They told us to lie face down and not speak, or otherwise they would kill us. It was very terrifying. Thinking about it makes me shiver.' Mr Hussain managed to escape after throwing a coffee table and called on his 35-year-old brother Tokeer to chase the three men down the road. Walid Salem was struck with a baseball bat after being knocked to the ground and suffered permanent brain injury. Mr Hussain and his brother were found guilty of causing grievous bodily harm.

Tokeer Hussain was jailed for thirty-nine months. The judge told the two men: 'If persons were permitted to take the law into their own hands and inflict their own instant and violent punishment on an apprehended offender rather than letting justice take its course, then the rule of law and our system of criminal justice, which are the hallmarks of a civilised society, would collapse.' Michael Wolkind, QC, defending Munir Hussain, said an appeal would be made. And it was. But it was public outrage that saw Mr Hussain released from prison in January. Three top judges at a Court of Appeal bowed to public pressure with the Lord Chief Justice Lord Judge saying calls for mercy had been 'intense and must be answered' and that the case was one of 'true exceptionality'. He added: 'Munir Hussain was acting under the continuing influence of extreme provocation. Involvement in this serious violence can only be understood as a response to the dreadful and terrifying ordeal and the emotional anguish which he had undergone. His family had effectively been kidnapped in their own home. He feared for their lives and the honour of his wife and daughter.' Mr Wolkind had told the court: 'I ask the court to reflect overwhelming public opinion in this case, not that Salem deserved what he got but that Munir does not deserve the sentence he was given. The court cannot deter a home-owner from responding in agony and despair.' Mr Hussain was allowed to walk free from Bullingdon Prison in Oxfordshire on January 20th 2010. He commented: 'I would like to thank everyone for their support. That support has been very comforting', but he added that the whole episode had left a 'sour taste'. His brother Tokeer had his thirty-nine month sentence reduced to two years but he had to remain in jail. Salem was the only intruder caught but his injuries meant he was not fit to plead when charged with false imprisonment. He has fifty past convictions and was later put in custody to await trial on an alleged credit card fraud.

The announcement in January 2010 that anthropologist, 42-year-old Dr Damian O'Doherty was going to live at Manchester

airport for a year doesn't really come under the banner 'politically correct' but it is laughingly wrong. For the cost of the
Government-funded experiment in which Dr O'Doherty lived
for up to eighteen hours a day for twelve months in terminals
and departure lounges to observe passengers' and workers'
habits, was estimated at around £40,000. The 'research' was
aimed at investigating how airports affect people – with the aim
of making them 'better places to visit or work' – and was paid
for by the Department of Business, Innovation and Skills. Said
Matthew Elliott, chief executive of the TaxPayers' Alliance: 'This
is a complete waste of money and shows just how out of touch
the Government is with views of tax-payers.' Dr O'Doherty
decreed it was serious research, however, saying: 'Some people
live in airports and 30,000 feet in the air. They commute from
place to place, have business meetings in an airport hotel and
then fly off somewhere else. I call them the "kinetic elite" –
always on the go, fixing business deals on their laptops, at the
same time talking on their iPhone and perhaps posting a Twitter
to friends and family. I've been researching airports for five
years and I just thought this would be the opportunity to experience airport life for myself. I enjoy sitting in the coffee shops
watching the hustle of airport life but I am spending a lot of time
shadowing project managers. I'm trying to think and act like
one.' Dr O'Doherty did not experience the misery of sleeping in
a departure lounge when flights are delayed for hours. He went
home to his family every night.

It was not what school trips are traditionally all about . . . the
division of 'haves' and 'have nots' with the 'haves' being
the ones who lost out. But that is what happened in Greater
Manchester when a trial Government-funded scheme across
Trafford Council in January 2010 offering lovely days out to
Knowsley Safari Park, training sessions at the Manchester
United football ground and visits to an indoor ski centre banned
children from well-off families but welcomed those who were
'economically disadvantaged'. Working parents were being

penalised, critics claimed. Even when parents offered to pay for their 'barred' children in the twenty-two schools in the pilot scheme, they were turned down. Said one: 'I'm really angry. I'm being penalised for working and wanting to do better for myself and my children. It's a nightmare. What sort of incentive does it give to these kids to want to go out and work if all their friends are allowed to go on fantastic trips but they aren't?' A spokesman for Trafford Council's Children and Young People's Service said it was a Government requirement that the funds be used to support children from the 'economically disadvantaged' families in the area. Those children receiving free school meals were the focus of the scheme as 'this ensures the funding goes to support children from lower-income families'. The Department for Children, Schools and Families said its guidance was 'crystal clear' and that 'no children should be left out. Activities should be available to all children – with those who can afford it being able to pay and take part . . . It is down to schools to use their professional judgements in deciding who is or is not eligible for subsidy.'

An investigation by the *Daily Express* uncovered dozens of eastern Europe-based websites which had branches in Britain offering advice on how to not only take advantage of our benefits system, but how to beat it too. The newspaper reported in January 2010 that the sites were helping to attract thousands of East European 'scroungers' to Britain. In Poland firms were signing up self-employed 'National Insurance tourists' for so-called consultancy jobs in our country while living in their home country and giving them advice on how to make the most of the health system and child welfare benefits. The firms also advertised that they could help negotiate bureaucratic red tape, applying on a client's behalf for child benefit, tax credit, maternity allowance and housing help, explaining about National Insurance numbers, emergency tax codes and the documents needed to claim benefit. One such firm, headed by businessman Ireneusz Klader, allegedly helped thousands of self-employed cab drivers, hairdressers and builders who live and work in Poland pay National Insurance in the UK. Said Klader: 'It's all entirely legal. They are working in consultancy jobs marketing my businesses by phone and internet and they are employed in the UK.' Under EU rules governing the free movement of peoples, these self-employed people can legitimately pay their National Insurance contributions in Britain. And if they contribute to the economy for the required length of time, then they are perfectly entitled to make a claim for state benefits, including the pension, if they have been paying long enough. The claiments received National Insurance and European health insurance cards. They could also try to claim child benefit and working tax credit because they were classed as low earners. Added Klader: 'Claiming such benefits requires the submission of forms that are dealt with by our specialists in London who have become highly experienced in handling Polish immigrants in Britain. We offer our clients help to claim only those benefits to which they are able to qualify, 100 per cent legally.' Not 100 per cent happy with the situation, Gerard Batten, UKIP MEP for London said: 'This just goes to show that when we sub-contract immigration policy to the EU we open ourselves to fraud. We must take back control of our borders.'

If your child returned home from their Church of England primary school and said that as well as Christianity they were being taught about other beliefs, you would hopefully welcome the diversity. For Islam, Judaism, Buddhism, Sikhism and Hinduism are now accepted as part of many schools' curriculum. But what about Jainism, Baha'i and Zoroastrianism? Yes, a mystery to most indeed. But in January 2010 these were three of the obscure religions ministers recommended that children as young as 5 should learn about. Said schools minister Diana Johnson: 'In 21st century Britain, it is vital that young people develop a good understanding of other people's beliefs, faiths and religions. This means learning about Christianity and other religions like Islam, Hinduism and Judaism, but also considering secular beliefs such as humanism and atheism.' All schools must teach Religious Education but it is not in the National Curriculum and councils have to gather together a Standing Advisory Council for Religious Education, made up of church leaders, teachers and subject experts to draw up syllabuses and oversee RE collective worship in schools. Schools watchdog Ofsted still complained that RE teaching was not rounded enough. In case you are wondering, followers of Zoroastrianism believe the dead should be eaten by vultures; Jains believe in non-violence and that animals and plants have souls, and the Baha'i faith teaches that all religions have valid origins and prohibits alcohol, drugs, adultery and party politics. Colin Hart, director of the Christian Institute described the primary school Religious Education programme as 'educational nonsense' and a 'multi-faith mish-mash'. He said: 'There are now even things that aren't religions at all such as humanism. If humanism is added, why not political beliefs? This will be a crook's tour of the most trivial aspects of faiths, so toned down that it will be how different religions use water and how they use light as a symbol. Things will be taken out of context and the integrity of each faith destroyed.'

In February 2010, well-known country expert Robin Page denounced the politically correct attitudes he said were letting wildlife predators flourish to the detriment of some of our best-loved wild animals and birds. Writing in the *Mail on Sunday* Page said political correctness had swept into the world of conserva-tion and was helping to kill the countryside 'A puritanical breed of wildlife fundamentalists now dominate official conservation,' he said. 'In their creed, nature is no longer red in "tooth and claw". Instead, it lives in a Disneyfied paradise in which Bambi and Thumper play at the feet of the Lion King as he feasts on croissants and soya milk.' Page expressed the opinion that preda-tors of the countryside were being granted the status of 'sainthood' while some of our most popular and vulnerable creatures are being decimated. 'These conservationists talk of nature finding its own "natural balance". What they forget, or fail to understand, is that the whole landscape of modern Britain is unnatural – wilderness has disappeared and the hand of man dominates. Consequently, to protect the weak and endangered, action has to be taken against the strong and numerous. In simple terms, this means controlling some of our rampant predators.' Page was prompted to speak out after the Royal Society for the Protection of Birds and the Government's wildlife quango Natural England announced it was going to release twenty young sea eagles a year in East Anglia over the next six years. Page said sea eagles had not lived or bred in England for hundreds of years and that the plan would endanger the lives of birds such as the tern, bittern, avocet and crane with full-grown sea eagles so large they can attack piglets, lambs and pet poodles. He also said that the lessening of tough treatment of predators had seen the numbers of certain species decline considerably. To further support his argument, Page quoted a Dr Ian Rotherham of Sheffield Hallam University who said that those wanting to control Britain's grey squirrel population was 'eco-xenophobia' adding of similar schemes: 'What's worse perhaps, is that they resonate with ideas growing with the BNP, and with other Right-wing groups across Europe.' Page concluded: 'Both Natural England and the RSPB are campaigning against largely imagined "wildlife crime". But the real crime is ignoring the effects of predation on our once common wildlife. It is time that honesty came into conservation, putting the welfare of our vulnerable species before bunny-hugging. Conserving our beautiful countryside should be about using common sense – not political correctness.'

You can imagine the frustration. You turn up at your local swimming pool for your usual Thursday morning session and find it is closed for 'training'. That is bad enough. But then you discover the pool was actually open – but only for female Muslim swimmers. Hull City Council was found out in February 2010 when some swimmers checked its website to see if the swimming pool timetable had been changed – and spotted an advert for the special Muslim swim sessions every Thursday morning between 10.30am and 12 noon. When tackled, the council admitted a session had taken place, but alongside staff training. It said the women were supervised by 'casual' staff while other employees 'do training or cleaning'. The swimmers were not convinced. Stormed one: 'If a group of Catholic women objected to using the pool when a group of Protestant women were swimming it would cause consternation. If these Islamic women had booked a private session why did the council not simply put up a sign saying "pool closed for private party" as they do for kids' birthdays? What makes this group any different from any other members of the community?' A council spokesman justified its actions by saying: 'The council is not providing a service that excludes non-Muslims but simply hiring a facility privately to a group who happen to be Muslim women. Other religious, social or cultural groups could do the same, subject to availability.'

If you were an employer, who would YOU choose? A job-seeker who was 'reliable' or one who was 'unreliable'? Recruitment boss 48-year-old Nicole Mamo tried to post an advert on her local Jobcentre Plus website for a £5.80 an hour NHS cleaner in Thetford, Norfolk. The ad seemed harmless enough: 'Domestic cleaner required immediately. A variety of different shifts available. Must be fluent in written and spoken English for health and safety reasons. Previous experience preferred. Training will be provided. Must be reliable and hard-working.' But when Ms Mamo called the Jobcentre the next day, she was told the ad could not go on screen as it discriminated against unreliable people. Said Ms Mamo: 'I laughed because I thought that was crazy. We supply the NHS with staff so it's very important for the patients that we have reliable workers. We find hundreds of temporary staff every week and are proud of our workers but our reputation is at stake if they aren't reliable.' Agreeing with Ms Mamo, a spokesman for the Plain English Campaign said:

'I am perplexed. It seems pretty plain English to me. I would have thought reliability for this sort of work is an important requirement. Have "unreliable" workers complained they are being discriminated against? Surely job discrimination is when an employer treats his employee in a negative or illegal manner. So how can highlighting positive traits be discriminatory? I'm afraid folly has overrun the world of common sense.' A spokesman for Work and Pensions said adverts for reliable applicants had not been banned and that Ms Mamo's advert did make it onto the Jobcentre website.

It has long been accepted that a young girl (or man – mustn't discriminate in this day and age) who wants to become a fully-fledged hairdresser starts off as a junior stylist while training. Well, in February 2010, the word 'junior' in a hair salon advert was criticised for discriminating against anyone who was not, well, 'junior'. It made Michelle Hilling, owner of U Hairdressing in the rather smart Newcastle suburb of Gosforth, cut up rough. It was the local Jobcentre Plus that refused to accept the advert unless Mrs Hilling dropped the word 'junior'. The word 'apprentice' was suggested as an alternative which Mrs Hilling unhappily had to agree to even though she felt the advert would then attract candidates with little hairdressing experience rather than someone who had had some training. She said: 'I have never come across anyone who was bothered about a job title like this. All I wanted was a junior stylist and even that proved to be wrapped in red tape. It doesn't matter what age they are. I've had a 45-year-old junior stylist before. The term has been used for years in hairdressing. The lady told me I couldn't use that term because it discriminated against old people. I explained that within the hairdressing industry the term is widely used and known. People working in the industry would know you don't have to be a teenager to be a junior stylist – it refers to your level of qualification.' The Department for Work and Pensions stood by the Jobcentre's decision, saying that such measures are essential to ensure employers don't fall foul of

Employment Equality Regulations which ban discrimination on the grounds of age when recruiting workers. None of this appeased Mrs Hilling who declared: 'This country has gone completely mad. Businesses are having to tread more and more carefully to avoid offending anyone. It is really quite offensive to suggest that someone older would be bothered by this.'

February that year was also the month when ANOTHER accusation of discrimination was made. This time it came from a 68-page report from the Equality and Human Rights Commission who said that girls wearing skirts to school may be breaking the law as it discriminated against transsexuals; the dress code may breach the rights of girls who feel compelled to dress as boys. The report noted that 'requiring pupils to wear gender-specific clothes is potentially unlawful' adding 'pupils born female with gender dysphoria experienced great discomfort being forced to wear stereotypical girls' clothes – for example a skirt'. The guidelines were produced in preparation for the Government's Equality Bill scheduled to come into force in autumn 2010 and which makes it a legal requirement for public authorities, including schools, to consider the impact on minority groups of all their policies — including how school uniforms might affect transsexual people. In short, schools have to ensure transsexual children do not suffer discrimination – or face potential legal sanctions. The Commission's official guidance, succinctly named Provision of Goods, Facilities and Services to Trans People – Guidance for Public Authorities in Meeting Your Equality Duties and Human Rights Obligations of – says schools have a duty to be 'proactive' in ensuring transsexual students are not discriminated against and that 'Uniform is a key issue for young trans people at schools. Many schools have strict uniform codes where boys and girls are required to wear particular clothes, for example, girls cannot wear trousers.' A spokesman from the Commission said: 'This is all about giving schools information which will help them interpret the law. It's about schools taking a bit of time to consider their policies, how flexible they are in accommodating pupils with different needs, and what they might need to do to both help pupils get the most out of school and potentially avoid situations which might culminate in difficult and costly legal action.' Although the Commission threatened to use 'costly legal action' on schools who fail to comply, many were thought to want to carry on with girls wearing skirts as part of their regulation school uniform. Retorted Elspeth Insch, head teacher of King Edward VI Handsworth School in Birmingham: 'The message is: not in my school. We're sticking with our skirts.' Added PC commentator Richard Littlejohn: 'I've no idea how many transsexual pupils there are at your average school. But I wouldn't have thought all that many . . . Surely any transsexual's sensitivities could be accommodated by a pair of slacks without making skirts a criminal offence? Of course, minorities' rights should be respected but not at the expense of criminalising the normal behaviour of the majority.'

An investigation in the *Mail on Sunday* on March 14th 2010 highlighted Britain's fall into the hands of discrimination laws which have us as the victims. The newspaper told how the company Forza AW, the biggest meat supplier to supermarket chain Asda, was turning away British workers at its production line in East Anglia because they did not speak Polish. Only Poles were accepted because they spoke the language fluently, with the company claiming it was because all health and safety training was conducted in Polish. A Polish version of the advert was also sent to several Eastern European shops in East Anglia with the words 'Work for Poles!' In short, it was a case of anti-British discrimination. The *Mail on Sunday* was alerted to an advert stressing that applicants 'must speak Polish' by a job-seeker and then listened in while he called recruitment agency OSR Recruitment who had posted it. Initially it said applicants had to be fluent in Polish, but wavered after several calls from the newspaper, saying the language requirement was 'not too important now'. Forza later claimed the advert was a mistake 'due to a breakdown in communications' and should never have gone out. The company is led by £780,000-a-year Max Hilliard, who was tackled by the newspaper. He said: 'We employ many English workers as well as Poles and Lithuanians, though I can't give you exact figures, and I assure you categorically that all our training and health and safety briefings are conducted in English, Polish or whatever the employee speaks . . . we would never turn down an English person for a job on the basis that they didn't speak Polish or any other language.' Mr Hilliard was right to make that point clear. For the company could have been breaking the law. Under the 1976 Equalities Act, unless there is a genuine need for a worker to speak a particular language it is against the law to require that they should do so as a condition of employing them. The *Mail on Sunday* carried a fierce leader. 'This country accepted laws against discrimination because they rightly put a stop to crude, cruel and unjust behaviour by employers and landlords. But from small beginnings, these measures have grown into a vast legal and bureaucratic apparatus, often heavy-handed and almost invariably politically correct. The suspicion has grown that this anti-discrimination industry is really meant to work in only one direction – that it is part of a huge effort to adapt Britain to immigration, rather than to help immigrants adapt to Britain.'

6

Health and Safety Gone Mad

The year 2009 heralded the great Wheelie Bin Controversy. Some said they were an eyesore; others that they were expensive. There were claims they were necessary to recycle waste and complaints that they were simply a waste of space. Local authorities said it was advice from the Health & Safety Executive which brought an end to the traditional dustbin and black refuse sacks. All in all, it was a right old mess. It was said that the real trouble was the 'over-zealous' rules inflicted on householders and the 'Big Brother' introduction of new style bins fitted with microchips, making it easier for the Government to introduce bin taxes on the amount of rubbish families produce. Some councils started charging £60 per household for the privilege of delivering the new bins. It was all a rather hysterical response to an EU directive that states Britain must drastically cut the amount of waste it sends to landfill by the year 2020. First there was a landfill tax of £32 per tonne (costing each household £25 a year). Then there was the waste 'allowance' given to local councils each year which was gradually reduced in a bid to beat too much rubbish going underground. If the councils did not come within this allowance they faced a fine of £180 per tonne.

Councils got anxious and started to act in strange ways. In Cumbria, a man found himself with a criminal record because he left his wheelie bin lid 4 inches open. In North Yorkshire, residents were asked to remove the inserts from their wheelie bins to prevent dustmen hurting their backs. In Wiltshire, householders found out that dustmen had been told not to move their wheelie bins if they couldn't pull them along with two fingers. A woman in Coventry found she was barricaded in her home by fifteen wheelie bins after she dared to complain about her dustmen. Rochdale council in Lancashire refused to empty the bin of arthritis sufferer, 64-year-old Mrs Patricia Pilkington because it was 12 inches from the pavement and therefore classed as 'not out for collection'. (It was later collected as a 'gesture of goodwill' – but only if the bin contained 'appropriate waste and has its lid closed . . .') A man in Blackburn called police after spotting two figures in his garden late at night. They turned out to be council officials checking for non-regulation dustbins. 'One woman in Henley-on-Thames said she would continue to use black refuse bags for her rubbish even if she faced the threat of being locked up. Keen gardener John Mason thought he was doing the right thing when he put bruised windfall apples in his garden waste wheelie bin only to be told they were not garden waste but had in fact 'contaminated' the bin. Officials at Flintshire County Council in North Wales said spoiled fruit like apples could have come from a kitchen and been in contact with uncooked meat resulting in the risk of bacteria. Said 64-year-old Mr Mason: 'It was sheer bureaucratic idiocy and really annoying.'

A health and safety manual issued in 2007 states that refuse collection involving plastic bags has 'potential for injury'. Another report said that dustmen (now called operatives) were likely to be injured by sharp objects in the bags, adding: 'The only risk (with wheelie bins) is during collection, and then only when they are overfull.'

Commented one critic of the imposed refuse collection scheme: 'The entire thing is a shambles. This Government is turning Britain into a police state . . .'

Many restrictive rules have been in force in nurseries and schools for some time. These include staff not being able to put sticking plasters or sun cream on children as both are too 'intrusive'. But the regulations are increasing – and getting more and more prohibitive. The year 2009 witnessed many of these: children having to wear goggles before handling Blu Tack modelling clay to prevent them rubbing the stuff in their eyes; the ban on making weird and wonderful creations from empty egg boxes in case of salmonella poisoning (and toilet rolls banned from similar model-making projects for health and hygiene reasons); teachers being given a 5-page document on the dangers of the solid glue Pritt Stick before being allowed to use it in their classrooms; staff barred from sending naughty children into the corridor because of potential fire hazard; no pictures allowed to hang in school below a height of 7ft; girls forbidden from wearing plastic hair bands because they could cause injury if there was a playground collision with another pupil; teachers required to take a bucket on school trips in case a child is sick; shaving foam no longer being used as a fun medium in art classes in case the children 'drown' in it; a three-legged race cancelled from one sports day because it is 'too dangerous'; PE lessons postponed because of wet grass; footballs, running, snowball fights and conker games banned from the playground unless they had some protection – in one instance, at Adlington Primary School in Macclesfield, pupils were ordered to wear safety goggles for a special conker contest being staged there, in case bits flew into their eyes. Said the school's head teacher Polly Broadhurst: 'We are quite an academic school and were determined the kids should have some fun – but we do it safely. In terms of wearing goggles we just considered it was better to be safe than sorry. Conkers are generally frowned on now because a child somewhere in the country, at some point, has been hurt playing a game.' She did admit, however, that 'I suppose it does really show that health and safety has gone over the top.' But the Health and Safety Executive said it was a myth that conker-bashing had been banned. Said a spokesman: 'This is one of the oldest chestnuts around, a truly classic myth. A well-meaning head teacher decided children should wear safety goggles to play conkers.

Subsequently some schools appear to have banned conkers on "health and safety" grounds or made children wear goggles, or even padded gloves! Realistically the risk from playing conkers is incredibly low and just not worth bothering about. If kids deliberately hit each other over the head with conkers, that's a discipline issue, not health and safety.' And did you know that there is actually a group called the Campaign for Real Conkers? One of their members, Keith Flett, had something to add to the conker danger debate. He said: 'There is a very small chance that a piece of conker might fly into your eye but you could get a piece of grit in your eye walking down the street – and you wouldn't wear goggles for that.' All these examples were cited in a survey of 600 British teachers as being in place to avoid injury and legal cases in today's 'compensation culture'. Commented Judith Hackitt, chairman of the Health and Safety Executive: 'These examples are frankly ridiculous. Health and safety is blamed for a lot of things not going ahead, but often they are about something else – high costs, an event that required a lot of organising or fear of being sued. Children cannot be wrapped in cotton wool; risk is part of growing up and our children need to learn how to manage risks in the real world.' And a spokesman for the Department for Children, Schools and Families commented: 'We urge schools to take a commonsense approach to keeping safe. Health and safety should not be a major burden and should not stop pupils from learning and playing. A small amount of risk is part and parcel of growing up and we do not subscribe to a cotton-wool culture of a sanitised childhood.'

Shortly after the survey, it was announced that schoolchildren at an average of ten schools a week were being ordered to wear clip-on ties instead of the traditional 'tie it yourself' ones. One school, the McAuley Catholic High School in Doncaster, brought in the uniform change after it was felt the pupils might accidentally be strangled during playtime games or set fire to their ties in science lessons. More than 400 pupils at the school signed a petition on the Facebook website calling for a return to their old school ties. Part of their rebellion was to accept the clip-on ties – but wear them on the lower buttons of their shirts . . .

In December 2008, it was revealed that primary schoolchildren were being taught how to blow their noses, including viewing a DVD telling them what to do if they had a cold. They were then asked to discuss their 'feelings' on hygiene and encouraged to look at a website sponsored by tissue company Kleenex at home with their parents. One parent of a child at Broad Oak Primary School in Manchester said the whole exercise was a 'waste of time' adding that 'I send my kids to school to learn, not for someone to show them how to blow their nose'. Defending the nose-blowing programme aimed at 5 to 11-year-olds, head teacher Sheila Marchant said: 'It is in the curriculum to teach children safe hygiene from an early age. And at this time of year there are many cold and flu bugs around.'

That same month, police officers who had for months managed to install roadside electronic speed indicators without a mishap were told they had to attend a health and safety seminar to ensure they could climb a ladder safely.

Around forty-five officers and over eighty civilian volunteers underwent the training organised by the police, Lancashire County Council and Lancashire Fire and Rescue. Said a frustrated senior police officer: 'It is a preposterous waste of police time and tax-payers' money and it is time the health and safety Gestapo had their wings clipped so that people can go about their jobs using their own common sense.'

As part of the seminar, the police and civilians were warned they must wear high-visibility jackets and leggings and cone off the area when installing signs in bad weather in case pedestrians bump into their ladder – which incidentally measures 3ft tall.

Explaining the need for the safety seminar, an official spokesman for Lancashire Police said: 'It would appear that, although working at less than 1 metre above ground level, staff should have been on a ladder training course. It is fair to say that risks associated with deployment of a speed indicator sign have not changed, but the risks associated with work at height were not fully appreciated initially.' The local council said the nine seminars already held had not cost anything – apart from staff time.

The last thing any emergency service has time to do on a call-out is put the paperwork in order first. But that is just what happened in January when coastguards throughout the country were ordered to fill out a health and safety questionnaire before responding to calls for help.

Under the new rules, issued by the Maritime and Coastguard Agency, the crews have to fill in the date and time of the call-out, the reason for the 'journey', any risks they might face en route and answer 'yes' or 'no' in answer to what action they have taken to ensure the risk is 'acceptable'.

All 400 of Britain's rescue units comprising 3,200 coastguard rescuers were affected by the new rules which even asked for details of risk from bad weather or sea currents. The latter is a strange question to pose considering the orders only apply to pre-journey risk assessments for coastguards using specially-equipped Land Rovers for land rescues. (The Maritime Agency is a branch of the Department of Transport.)

Commented one coastguard: 'When we were first told about this, we simply couldn't believe it. When we get a call asking us to go out and rescue someone we need to go there without delay. But they are asking us to waste time in the office filling out this stupid form. Also, none of us really knows what we are realistically meant to fill in. I mean, how are we meant to know what risks there might be before we get there? And do they expect us to get a full weather forecast before we go out? It's ridiculous. All we want to do is save lives. The impression we get is that the bosses are doing everything they can to make sure their hands are legally clean if there is any kind of problem.'

In November 2008, coastguards were told that they can no longer use flares during night-time rescues as they could 'cause considerable injury . . .'

It might sound self-explanatory; Cadbury's Dairy Milk chocolate is likely to contain milk. But just to reinforce the fact, Cadbury's started putting a picture of a glass of milk being poured into a chocolate chunk on its wrappers in January 2009. It also explained that there is 'the equivalent of three quarters of a pint of milk in every half pound of milk chocolate'. And just in case a chocolate-eater with an allergy to milk missed these warnings, there were warnings in capital letters in yellow boxes announcing the choccy bar 'Contains Milk'. The famous chocolate company did similar with its Dairy Milk Whole Nut bars ('Contains Nuts, Milk') and mentioned the nut content four times. A company spokesman said: 'We are meeting legal requirements. We want people to know that allergens are listed clearly.' But commented Moira Austin, of the Anaphylaxis Campaign, a support group for allergy sufferers: 'I can understand why people would think the world had gone mad.' Ms Austin was probably not surprised to hear that later that month supermarket Asda put a warning on its plastic milk bottles that milk was contained therein. It later removed the warnings saying: 'To be consistent we always state the allergens in a product irrespective of whether it is a single ingredient or not. But everyone knows milk is milk.' January was also the month that the Happy Egg Company put the warning 'Contains eggs' on its egg-filled boxes.

Bishop Jonathan Blake came up with a heavenly idea for his sons' school project. When the lads were told they had to be photographed reading in an unusual place, the Most Rev Blake put 8-year-old Nathan and 7-year-old Dominic atop his 40ft chimney and took their picture. But neighbours of the Blake family in Welling, south-east London, thought the Bishop's actions in February were one hell of a risk to the boys and called the police. Officers came and arrested 52-year-old Mr Blake and his 49-year-old wife on suspicion of neglect. Mr Blake, Bishop of Greater London for the Open Episcopal Church, later said he was kept in a blood-stained cell overnight and said he would launch a claim for false imprisonment, adding: 'My family were traumatised. The children were weeping as they watched their father being frogmarched to a police van.' This despite one neighbour describing the roof-top performance as 'bonkers' and asking the question 'Why would you ever dream of putting your kid on the chimney?' Mr Blake insisted the boys had both worn harnesses and were used to adventure sports and rock-climbing.

Police said they would take no further action against Mr Blake.

It seemed a 'wheely' good challenge – two BBC Radio Essex presenters seeing who could change a car tyre the fastest as part of the BBC's Big Skill initiative in March. But it was not enough for Christine Penhall and Graham Bannerman to receive instructions from a qualified mechanic before embarking on the fun competition. First a risk assessment had to be drawn up and health and safety forms filled in. Then an ambulance complete with first-aider and a paramedic was called to be on stand-by in case the presenters had an accident handling 'unfamiliar equip-ment'. Said Caroline Lake, the mechanic who demonstrated how a tyre could safely be changed: 'All we were doing was taking off a couple of wheels. Yet we had to have medical experts there in case something went wrong. It was just barmy and silly.' A BBC spokesman said they had just ensured there was 'a basic precaution' in place with the two voluntary St John Ambulance medics 'to administer any basic first-aid require-ments'.

Following on from lessons in nose-blowing for children, teachers were invited to attend courses on 'effective hand-washing' in April. The course – with the title The Importance of Hand-Washing in Schools – was organised by the borough of

Newham in East London and offered places for twenty-three teachers of personal, social and health education to learn 'to make sure hot and cold running water, soap and drying facilities are available'. They were also briefed on how proper hand-washing can help 'individuals achieve a higher state of body image'. Speaking at his Brighton College's annual education conference, head Mr Richard Cairns said: 'Hand-washing matters and children do indeed need to be told from time to time to wash their hands regularly. But do twenty-three teachers need to come out of school to be taught for two-and-a-half hours about how to use water, soap and drying facilities to improve pupils' body image? What saddens me most about all this is that money that could have gone to pay a teacher will instead go to pay a "professional developer".'

Potholes in a road in the village of Smalley, near Derby, prevented folk from getting their post for a week in May. That was because Royal Mail took exception to the fact that one of their van drivers had jarred his back after driving over one of the holes. It sent out letters saying mail would not be delivered to Bell Lane until the pothole was filled in. Strangely, although normal mail was not distributed, the letters announcing the ban were hand-delivered. They came from local delivery officer Ruth Rowe and informed the residents that the postman was now off sick and 'I have suspended delivery of mail to your address until this problem is rectified. I am very sorry for any inconvenience caused but I have to consider the safety of my employees and also possible damage to our vehicle.' The potholes were filled in and service resumed as normal, but said one villager: 'The potholes were only three inches deep. I've never damaged myself or my car in eight years of driving down the lane.' Added another: 'If it wasn't for the date on the letter, I'd have thought it was an April Fools' joke.'

Little Daniel Johnson was barred from building pebble dams in a local stream in case he sparked a flash flood. That was in May when Terry Williams, chairman of the Parish Council of Nettleham, near Lincoln, declared: 'We can't have people doing this sort of thing willy-nilly. We are very concerned about the potential consequences of flooding.' Daniel, 6, and his father Rob, 33, were warned that the pebble piles could block the 2-inch high stream and cause a 'major disaster'. Said a perplexed Rob: 'I am gobsmacked by this, it's ridiculous. We have made a pebble dam a few times. It's the stuff you do with your kids.' The council letter berated Mr Johnson and his little boy for 'repeatedly rebuilding dams' after the council had cleared the 5-inch piles away and ordered that 'you cease your activity forthwith'. To be fair, parts of Nettleham were flooded in June 2007, but before that the last flood was in the winter of 1947–48 and it is hardly likely a handful of pebbles would cause a major disaster. Said one villager: 'It does seem a little like political correctness gone mad that a little boy can't put a few pebbles in a brook . . .'

Thousands of tourists flock to the famous cathedral town of Canterbury, Kent, every year. For them, the sense of history of the place, combined with an excellent university, good restaurants and extensive shopping opportunities all make the place very much worth a visit. The fact that Canterbury did not cater to homosexuals probably did not cross their minds. But it certainly crossed the minds of the campaign group Pride in Canterbury who criticised the city as a 'cultural wilderness' because it had no gay bar and did not extend a fulsome welcome to the gay community as a whole. Said spokesman Andrew Bretell: 'We do not believe the council wants a thriving lesbian, gay, bisexual and transgender community in our city. They're more interested in ticking their equality boxes than they are in dealing with the real gay issues . . . the area doesn't send out an image that it's OK to be gay.' The council's chief executive, Colin Carmichael, refuted the claim, saying that the council had provided Pride in Canterbury with more than £4,000 of funding since 2005 'to help them identify the needs of the gay community and promote their concerns'. Commented a local stall-holder: 'I can't imagine a gay American bloke saying "Well, I'd love to see one of the most beautiful cathedrals in the world, but let's go somewhere else because there is no gay bar . . ."'

The weekly trip by 72-year-old George Pretty to pick up fish and chips for fellow residents at a sheltered housing unit took a battering in June when health and safety barminess slapped a ban on him because he did not carry home the lunch in an insulated box. Housing wardens at the Lakenham Fields complex in Norwich said there was a risk of food poisoning because the fish might get cold on the three-minute drive back. A notice was even pinned up explaining to the residents that the fish and chip lunch had had to be cancelled 'due to health and safety reasons'. Said Mr Pretty: 'We were told that we had to have boxes like the ones used for meals on wheels as the food has to be kept at a certain temperature. But all the orders are wrapped individually in polystyrene boxes and would be eaten only five minutes after I picked them up. Everyone used to say how lovely and hot they were. It's bureaucracy and the world gone mad.' The eighteen residents chipped away at the order and successfully had it overturned after involving the local press. And Norwich City Council entered the fray to say that external health and safety advice had been rather over-zealously applied. A spokesman said the ban had been introduced with the 'best intentions' and added: 'The council's own food safety experts do not think there is a health risk to residents having lunch in this way and our advice is that there is no problem in continuing their weekly fish and chips . . .'

Oh, the joys of picking strawberries on long, hot summer days! And the PYO (Pick Your Own) invitation is always readily taken up. Accidents doing so have never been recorded for there is little harm that can befall one meandering among the rows of strawberries. Not so, declared health and safety officials who ordered one of Britain's biggest strawberry farms to install walkways, handrails and bridges and cordon off potholes after carrying out a risk assessment following the fall of an elderly visitor. It would be funny if it was not so serious. For in June Boddington's Berries in Mevagissey, Cornwall said it now had to close because of the demand to 'radically refurbish' its 20-acre farm. Said owner, 45-year-old Phil Boddington: 'To us it's a pick-your-own farm but to insurers and the health and safety people it's a strawberry factory. It's a sad day when a pick-your-own farm is closing because of health and safety fears.'

Mr Boddington said that only two people had been injured in the forty years the PYO had been running. Unfortunately, in this 'claim culture' the last one was an elderly lady who filed a claim against the farm's insurers over a fall that left her in hospital. 'With that claim, our insurance premium more than doubles. It was already in the thousands of pounds and that was far too much.'

It might read 'Welcome' but that mat outside your front door could just be looking to trip you up. At least that is what Stoke City Council decided in June when it told tenants to remove not only the welcome mats but also pot plants and carpets from porches outside their flats in case they caused people to fall during a fire evacuation. The rules applied to council flats with communal areas and the council said tenants were welcome to put items inside their homes BEHIND their front doors. One tenant, 53-year-old Annette Ball who was told to remove a doormat, table and chair, commented: 'We've tried to make our porches homely, but we're not even allowed to have a picture on the wall . . . but we're forced to leave our rubbish in bags on stairwells twice a week and that's more dangerous.'

It was a case of men getting high-handed over high heels when in August the Trade Union Congress declared that stiletto shoes should be banned from the workplace because they are not only a health and safety hazard, but sexist too. The predominantly male group insisted that women should wear 'sensible shoes' with heels no more than an inch high to prevent back injury and falling over. In short, they decreed, high-powered jobs should not necessitate high-heeled shoes, adding: 'Congress believes high heels may look glamorous on the Hollywood catwalks but are completely inappropriate for the day-to-day working environment.' It even, published a safety guide detailing 'heels should have a broad base and be no higher than 4cm (1.5in) . . . If worn for long stretches, no higher than 2cm (0.8in).' Women, of course were furious. Said Tory MP Nadine Dorries: 'The TUC need to get real, and stop using overtly sexist tactics by discussing women's stilettos to divert attention away from Labour chaos.'

There was a loss of colour at Ferndown Carnival in Dorset in July when the council decreed that traditional bunting could no longer be hung from lampposts. The reasoning behind this was that the weight from a string of flags might bring the lampposts down. Said Rod Maidstone, lighting engineer at Dorset County Council: 'Internal corrosion, which cannot be seen, may have weakened the column and the additional load could lead to it collapsing.' There was also the concern that the bunting could 'sag and become entangled in passing buses or lorries'.

Carnival organiser Jane Harding, 42, was stunned at the decision saying it was health and safety gone mad, adding: 'It's absolutely ridiculous. The bunting is lightweight plastic. It doesn't sag or get heavier when it gets wet and it's designed to be strung up like this. If the lampposts can't take the weight, it makes you wonder whether they should be up at all.' Ferndown was not alone as a victim of the thought police. The city council in Dundee banned schoolchildren from selling home-made cakes at school fêtes on health and safety grounds (backing down only after 'further consideration of available risk mitigation measures' – and being the subject of public ridicule). In Cumbria, the Brampton Cottage Hospital garden party was moved after twenty years, on the grounds that visitors might seek shelter in the hospital if it rained and pose a risk of infection. And in Longhope, Gloucestershire, where the village fête was celebrating its 90th year, signs publicising the event were removed because they were not authorised by the local Highways Agency. A similar fate faced a primary school fête in Bromley, Kent, when it was told it faced prosecution unless it removed 'unauthorised advertisements' for the event.

There was a ban on parents at the East Beds School Sports Partnership Athletics Day in July amid fears that a paedophile might sneak into the event and abduct a child.

Hence, there were no mums and dads cheering the 270 children along at the event which is the highlight of the sports season for pupils at four primary schools in the villages of Biggleswade and Sandy in Bedfordshire. Organisers made their decision after a risk assessment – the bane of anyone trying to plan an activity nowadays when in the past there has simply been no need. They said they could not prevent 'unsavoury' characters getting into the grounds of the host school and could not guarantee the children's safety. Justifying the decision, Paul Blunt, development manager of East Beds School Sports Partnership said the 'ultimate fear' was that a child could have been abducted at the event, adding: 'If we let parents into the school they would have been free to roam the grounds. All unsupervised adults must be kept away from children.'

Parents said it was health and safety gone mad and that although there should be measures to protect children, common sense 'must prevail'. The ban also brought comment from the Campaign for Real Education with its chairman Nick Seaton stating: 'It's totally unreasonable to ban parents from a sports day. It's a serious misjudgement. If you followed this thinking you wouldn't be able to let your child out of the front door.' Sadly, this was not an isolated case. In Devon, parents were stopped from taking photographs of their children at sports day in case the pictures turned up on unsavoury internet sites.

* * *

The Severn Vale housing society banned children from a communal paddling pool at Crouch Court, Tewkesbury, Gloucestershire, in July because it said it was too dangerous.

The plug was pulled on the pool when health and safety enthusiasts said it was a 'significant drowning hazard' as it was left unattended at night and a child could get hurt.

The inflatable 10ft-wide pool was less than 2ft deep and had been a permanent fixture since 2005. Youngsters were supervised by adults, including a trained lifeguard.

Said one disgruntled parent, 42-year-old Helen Crozier, responsible for maintaining the pool: 'They say that if I don't move it immediately they will. We can't man it 24/7 but there's always someone supervising the kids and my boyfriend is a trained lifeguard. I'm so upset, I've been in tears. I'm so disappointed for the kids.' Commented Tewkesbury Conservative MP Laurence Robertson: 'Unfortunately it seems the paddling pool has become another victim of the tragic blame culture.'

Sunday, July 19th saw one giant picnic throughout Britain as part of the Eden Project's The Big Lunch and aimed at drawing neighbours and communities closer together. Businessman Ian Blackwell, 63, was just one of the 7,000 volunteer organisers and had gone to a lot of trouble to plan his picnic on Castle Meadow, Totnes, Devon. But he was taken aback to be asked by Totnes Town Council to take out insurance of a staggering £5m. The council clerk, David Edwards, said the insurance was to protect organisers who put on events on council-owned land. 'They have responsibility for the event and the land,' he said. 'Should anybody have an accident they will be personally liable for that injury and I am sure they don't want that.' But retorted Mr Blackwell: 'It just seems ludicrous in a public field that's fenced off,' he said. 'We're not having a BBQ or music. The worst that can happen is somebody's going to choke on a chicken bone or get stung by a wasp.' Nevertheless, Mr Blackwell paid the £70 to obtain the insurance cover – even though, as he rightly pointed out, if he had been organising a birthday party in the park for friends and family alone, 'we're apparently then not responsible for their actions . . .'

Swimming a goodly number of lengths at your local pool is excellent exercise and a rewarding measure of your stamina in the water. Somehow, swimming a length or two does not match up. But Barking and Dagenham Council which runs Dagenham Swimming Pool in Essex banned swimmers in July from covering lengths for health and safety reasons. Swimming widths, they said, made it easier for lifeguards to ensure pool-users' safety. The municipal pool is 33.3 metres long (108ft) and 25 metres wide (85ft) and is safely used by thousands of swimmers every week but the council decreed the swimming lanes should now run widthways rather than lengthways. Said a council spokesman: 'This enables people who are less confident to swim lengths of the shallow end to help them get fit and also it makes it easier to see where people are swimming and what they are doing. It's about variety, giving a whole host of swimming options.' Commented one regular pool-user, 33-year-old Dean Bradford: 'A lot of elderly people swim lengths of the pool to maintain their stamina and health and young people swim lengths to become better swimmers. There are also those people who swim lengths as part of a training regime to compete in the sport . . . This is just the nanny state gone mad. It's just another obstacle for people trying to get fit and healthy.'

The good people of Helston in Cornwall at first thought it was a wind-up. They had heard that 63-year-old church warden Roger Nott was no longer allowed to keep the church clock ticking over because of health and safety reasons. Volunteer Mr Nott, who had had the job of winding the clock mechanism at the top of St Michael's church for three years without doing himself any harm, was told it was too dangerous a task – even though someone had safely done so for over 200 years. Said Mr Nott:

'To wind the clock up is a simple operation carried out up a ladder and involves reaching out from the top in order to reach the winding mechanism. I take five or six steps up the ladder. I'm not bothered about the height. My predecessor retired when he was 82 and he still managed it fine.' The warden was banned from manually keeping the clock going on the advice of the Truro Diocesan Guild of Ringers who said health and safety was a key issue. A spokesman said: 'Unfortunately, many people who wind clocks up aren't getting any younger and their safety is important.'

In case you are wondering if the clock at St Michael's was to stop ticking for the first time since 1793, parishioners hoped to solve the problem by fitting a £5,000 automatic winding system.

It is normally a police officer who offers the advice 'Mind how you go . . .' But in the case of West Midlands Police it was the lawmen themselves who were given advice on taking care. For they were warned that slippery customers don't just come in the form of villains – but soggy, fallen autumn leaves too. The 'seasonal danger' campaign was aimed at police officers treading tentatively to avoid tripping over. They were also told to take care when driving on icy roads in winter and to watch out for sudden rainfall in spring. Summer too, can hold danger for our boys in blue – with a warning to beware of bright sunshine. The guidelines were made public in October 2009 for incredibly, a police Personnel Committee report revealed that the number of accidents involving officers had rocketed from 787 between 2002 and 2003 to 1,422 in 2008 to 2009. Just what on earth causes them so many mishaps? A spokesman for West Midlands Police said that slips, trips and falls made up 23 per cent of total accidents among its officers in autumn and winter and 17 per cent in spring and summer. He added: 'As the primary causation factor, it is incumbent on the force to take action to reduce the numbers of injuries occurring from these incidents.' But commented one officer: 'We do not need to be told that bright sunshine can affect your vision, that rain, ice and snow can make underfoot conditions slippery or that rain makes you wet. This is absolutely ludicrous and whoever came up with such a brainwave should be sacked.' This view was supported by the West Midlands Police Federation whose chairman, Andy Gilbert noted: 'While we welcome anything that enhances officer safety, there is a clear danger here of being patronising and stating the obvious. No-one has ever come to me and said "I have been injured because no-one told me it was going to rain" or that "the sun would get in my eyes . . . "'

A school's 'healthy eating' policy seemed a half-baked idea when it prevented 9-year-old Olivia Morris sharing her birthday cake with fellow pupils. Olivia was allowed to blow out the candles on the cake which was lovingly made by her great-grandmother but then she had to take it home. Cake simply did not comply with the healthy living message at Rockingham Infant and Junior School in Rotherham whose head teacher Heather Green insisted that although 'we love celebrating the birthdays of our pupils in class and in assemblies, at the same time, however, we are working really hard to promote healthy eating and lifestyles among our pupils. It is a tricky balance not to give a mixed message to pupils if we say to them "eat healthily at school" but at the same time we say "bring in cakes and buns to celebrate all our different events". We also take into account children with allergies and the pressure some parents feel they are under to provide such treats.' Great-grandma, 79-year-old Eileen Morris, who has been baking cakes for her family to take to school for forty years or so, felt the ban was 'crazy' and said: 'I understand the need to teach children healthy eating but surely a birthday cake is a special treat.' The cake ban controversy was not helped by the fact that TV cook Jamie Oliver launched his healthy-eating campaign 'Ministry of Food' in Rotherham. The not having your cake nor eating it dictat cropped up later that year in Hertfordshire when the Friends of Royston Hospital refused to accept five trays of cakes donated by exercise club, the Royston Runners. It had been the tradition for twenty-four years that the running fundraisers gave cakes as their 'entry fee' to an annual 10km fun run and afterwards auctioned off some to raise funds for the hospital. Any still left over were given to patients. But this time around, the 'Friends' of the hospital said they could not accept the cakes because they did not know under what conditions they had been made. They were also concerned that diabetic patients may 'accidentally' eat them and become ill. A hospital spokesman said that the runners would have to have their kitchens inspected before the cakes – or indeed any food – could be accepted because 'we just don't know where it comes from'. Chairman of the Royston Runners, 64-year-old Maurice Hill commented: 'I feel sorry for the patients because they don't get much pleasure. Many of them are old and very, very ill and so they enjoy receiving our cakes each year.'

Retired radio producer David France and his wife Katie felt they were doing doubly good for the environment in one go: not only were they taking their scrap metal to an official recycling dump, but they were walking there too. But after arriving at the site in Blandford, Dorset, the couple were told they could not go in on . . . yes, you've guessed it . . . health and safety grounds . . . because they might get run over. That meant Mr France had to leave his wife at the gate keeping guard over the scrap metal while he walked the 400 yards home to get his car. He said: 'It was farcical. I thought we were being doubly green by taking our recycling there on foot.' A spokesman for the RAC Foundation said the incident was 'bonkers' adding: 'Short car journeys are more harmful in terms of carbon dioxide emissions.' Dorset County Council later said that walk-in recyclers will be allowed into the dump – but only after a safety warning.

It was eggxactly the kind of health and safety approach that makes you feel like cracking up. Professor Susannah Eykyn keeps twenty-nine hens at her home in Minterne Parva, near Dorchester, Dorset, who are all highly productive in the egg department. In fact so productive that Professor Eykyn gave lots away to friends and family. Even then, there were eggs galore, so she thought it was a good idea to approach the owner of the village shop and ask if some could be sold there. She was told a licence to do so was required from DEFRA – the Department for Environment, Food and Rural Affairs. So Professor Eykyn called the department. First a DEFRA inspector called round, at one point donning a protective suit to look inside the hen hut during the three-hour visit. Then there was a visit by an Environmental Health officer (who also stayed for three hours) who wanted to know what Professor Eykyn cleans her kitchen with. She was also told how to clean and weigh an egg properly and, even though her egg-buying public are likely to all live close by, she had to make the egg boxes with a code identifying the 'establishment, origin and method of production'. It was only after Professor Eykyn filled out a pile of paperwork that her kitchen was officially declared a DEFRA-approved packing station and she was declared a 'business manager' authorised to sell eggs. Said Professor Eykyn: 'It does seem to be quite remarkable that for me to sell a few surplus eggs at the village store I needed to be subjected to this utter nonsense. The inspector had to drive from wherever he was based to come and inspect my home and treat me like a child. I mean, where are we at in this country? These jobsworth people don't seem to differentiate between someone like me who has a few extra eggs to sell and someone who supplies Tesco with 100,000 a year.' A spokesman for DEFRA explained that 'traceability is important for human and animal health, as well as enforcing marketing regulations. People have a right to know where their food comes from and that it's safe.' It really was a case of teaching your granny how to, well, suck eggs. For Professor Eykyn is an authority on bacterial diseases.

When it comes to the rather innocuous leisure activity of bowling, the Health and Safety Executive certainly did not strike a happy chord. It compiled a report released in November 2009 that made the fun sport sound rather deadly, with the conclusion that ten-pin bowling alleys throughout the country constitute a 'very dangerous' environment for families, with the high possibility of children or teenagers running down the bowling lanes and getting trapped in the skittle pick-up and set-up machinery at the end of the 60-foot lanes. It also pointed out that if a bowler was suddenly overcome with an urge to walk down the lane and knock the pins down by hand, that too presented a dangerous situation. Staff were ordered to wear earmuffs to stifle the noise of balls hitting the pins. Even more ludicrous was the suggestion of putting barriers across lanes because it meant bowlers would not actually be able to see what they were aiming for . . . This suggestion (together with the others) was later withdrawn because 'customers need to see the pins and bowling balls entering the machine, managing the risk of access into the machine from the lanes is more difficult'. It instead told bowling alley operators to fit photoelectric beams to lanes so the pin-setting machines will cut off automatically if someone 'trespasses' on the alley. None of the accidents the Health and Safety Executive was out to prevent have ever actually occurred (though to be fair, it was compiled after a technician was crushed to death in 2006 at a London bowling alley when a pin-setting machine was left plugged in). The report took two years to complete and cost £250,000. An HSE spokesman backed their report by saying: 'The investigation revealed that the machinery used nationally in bowling alleys did not have adequate safety features.' But John Ashbridge of the Ten-Pin Bowling Proprietors Association (amazing just what organisations are out there!) was not impressed. He had witnessed HSE inspectors examining a bowling centre and found their determination to label such places as dangerous, 'hilarious'. He said: 'I have been in this industry for forty years and I have never known any member of the public injured by a bowling pin-setter. I have never heard of anyone going near the pins.' Over to our favourite insanely politically-correct opposers, the TaxPayers' Alliance, who commented: 'The HSE has overreacted to a one-off tragedy by wasting a fortune of tax-payers' money producing a pointless, navel-gazing report . . .'

Remember those days of chivalry when many a male hand would reach out and offer to help a young mum struggling to manoeuvre a pram up a flight of stairs? Well, in those days, such aid could be offered without insurance! Nowadays, of course it is all so, so different. Travelling alone with her 10-week-old baby Oliver, 26-year-old Vicky Pachner asked for assistance at her local train station in Wadhurst, East Sussex. She was refused because staff said they were not insured to do so, with a spokesman for Southeastern Trains adding that another main factor in the refusal was that staff may have thought their time out to help would affect the safe running of trains. Mrs Pachner, who had been on the way to a routine hospital check-up on her son, was quite rightly not impressed. She said: 'I asked the lady behind the counter if someone could help me carry the buggy up the stairs and down the steps on the other side to reach the platform. She said no-one was available to help so I asked if she could or the other man in the ticket office with her. It's only a small village station so it's not as if they were rushed off their feet and really busy. Then the lady said they could not help because they were not insured to lift things like prams.' It was a fellow woman passenger who then came to Mrs Pachner's aid. The first-time mum sent a letter of complaint to Southeastern Trains after the incident in October 2009. They replied saying they might have been able to help if she had removed baby Oliver from the buggy and collapsed it. To add insult, Mrs Pachner's husband went to the same station a few days after the incident and WAS helped to carry the buggy by a different member of railway staff . . .

When the train on which 58-year-old Chris Haynes was travel-ling back home to London after a day out at Newbury Racecourse in Berkshire broke down and it was announced all passengers could get a free drink on board as compensation, he headed straight to the buffet car. Noticing egg sandwiches on sale, Mr Haynes requested if he might purchase some. He was told he couldn't for health and safety reasons because, explained the steward: 'Don't you see? If the train has to be evacuated you could choke to death on the sandwich.' Mr Haynes, a bar manager, and therefore probably acquainted with the potential dangers of sandwich-eating was rather taken aback, retorting later: 'I've never, ever heard anything so ludicrous in all my life. There was a queue of people behind me and they all looked shocked . . . I said I didn't understand how health and safety came into selling a hungry stranded passenger an egg sandwich on a broken-down train.' A spokesman for First Great Western said she was not aware of the sandwich-refusal incident, adding: 'It is not our policy to refuse to serve customers on these grounds.' Mr Haynes arrived back at Paddington hungry and two and a quarter hours late.

One wonders if it was really necessary, but Warwickshire County Council (in conjunction with the NHS, Age Concern Warwickshire and other local 'partners' including Warwickshire County Council's PHILLIS (Promoting Health and Independence through Low Level Integrated Support) Service, Warwickshire County Council Mobile Libraries and Library Home Delivery Service, Healthy Living Network, Orbit Care and Repair, Rugby Carers and Brunswick Healthy Living Centre) obviously thought it was. The problem was dangerous slippers and the threat to the elderly of falling out of them or indeed while in them. Hence, in November 2009, the council announced its county-wide scheme to replace old slippers with new £5 footwear boasting 'non-slip soles, good support and a Velcro fastening to ensure a snug and tailored fit'. The scheme also offered 'falls-prevention' advice such as although wide fittings were also available 'it is imperative that slippers are tried on to make sure the fit is right'. The council further added that 'Although slipper service schemes have worked well in smaller areas of the county, the council was keen to provide an equitable service for all Warwickshire residents aged 50+.' Slippers would be available at PHILLIS events and a small selection on sale at mobile libraries and home visits were offered. Warwickshire County Council felt that between 20 to 30 per cent of falls could be prevented and that badly-fitting slippers 'significantly increase the risk of an older person falling at home'. Commented Councillor Colin Hayfield, the council's Portfolio Holder for Adult Social Care: 'This simple but effective measure is helping to prevent falls and accidents around the home.'

Oh, let us believe that when Australian public health expert Dr Nathan Grills assessed the 'negative impact' of Father Christmas' 'image' in the British Medical Journal, it was all just a bit of tongue-in-cheek Ho, Ho, Ho. Dr Grills criticised Santa for a multitude of sins; his 'rotund sedentary image' because it 'equates obesity with cheerfulness' for one. Remarked Dr Grills: 'To create a supportive environment for Santa's dieting we should cease the tradition of leaving him cookies, mince pies, and milk, brandy or sherry. This is bad not only for Santa's waistline but for parental obesity. When Santa is full, dad is a willing helper. Santa might also be encouraged to adopt a more active method to deliver toys – swapping his reindeer for a bike or walking or jogging.' Dr Grills also said giving Santa alcohol at every port of call was not good either as it could give him drink problems and encourage him to be a drink-driver (of his sleigh). Added Dr Grills (and yes, we think he WAS taking the mickey out of mad political correctness): 'Other dangerous activities that Santa could be accused of promoting include speeding, disregard for road rules and extreme sports such as roof-surfing and chimney-jumping.'

'Health and safety gone mad' is a popular refrain of today's modern world. And that is exactly what 57-year-old Linda Langford said when she was ordered to remove two garden gnomes from outside the door of her flat in Tipton, West Midlands. The 6-inch gnomes had happily stood there in the passageway for nine years without causing harm or complaint. But then the local Sandwell Council decreed they could cause people to trip over if trying to escape from a fire. Miss Langford, incidentally, was also ordered to remove her doormat and a welcome plaque on the passageway wall. To be fair to the council, it was acting on a new policy on items outside flats following a review of safety issues provoked when a fire in Camberwell, south London, earlier that year had claimed the lives of six people. Said council spokesman Mahboob Hussain: 'I have personally received complaints about items blocking communal areas. In some extremes, I have seen people blocking hallways in a manner that is just not acceptable.' Mr Hussain changed his point of view when the council later said the gnomes could stay and said the policy has been 'misinterpreted', adding: 'As long as there is not an excessive number of gnomes or similar items in communal areas, and as long as there isn't a problem with these items being damaged through anti-social behaviour they can stay.' Miss Langford still felt it was a case of health and safety gone mad, saying: 'The idea that my two little gnomes are a fire hazard or that they are dangerous in any way is absolutely ridiculous.'

Officials of Coventry City Council were out in force after Christmas armed with tape measures to check that wheelie bins were not overfull with rubbish and thereby prompting lids to gape and possible injury to refuse collectors. If a lid was a quarter of an inch open then the bin was not collected. It was feared falling rubbish may hurt the dustmen. Said one householder: 'The bin men have passed us by. They've emptied my neighbour's bin but haven't touched ours just because it is open a bit. There are another forty bins I can see on this road that they haven't emptied. It's pathetic.' Extra bags left out with rubbish were not collected either, with families told to take them to the tip or wait until the refuse collectors were ready to collect them.

The measuring measures and the rubbish risk in general were explained by Coventry City councillor Hazel Noonan. She said: 'It's for health and safety reasons and spillage reasons that we don't collect extra items. There is concern that spillage can occur as over-filled bins or bags are taken from the pavement to the road and injure people standing there. We have to be careful.'

Stalwart observer of and commentator on political correctness gone off the rails, Richard Littlejohn of the *Daily Mail* in February 2010 reported how one of his readers, Morag Faulds, was stopped from carrying her newborn son along a corridor at the Royal Alexandra Hospital in Paisley, Scotland because she might drop him. The midwife said the child should instead be wheeled in a crib. Commented Littlejohn: 'Elf'n'Safety, you understand, even though mothers have been carrying babies for millennia.' That same day, he told how pallbearers refused to carry a coffin at a funeral because the footpath leading to the church was uneven and produced a trolley to carry it instead. The mourners protested and offered to carry the coffin themselves. 'Just two examples proving there's no escape from the Nanny State, from the cradle to the grave,' noted Littlejohn.

Organisers of the Whitsun Cheese-Rolling event were always aware there were a few minor injuries in the rough and tumble of the competition in which a 7lb wheel of Double Gloucester could reach speeds of up to 70mph. But they still thought the health and safety 'police' were a little crackers to make them cancel the chasing of the mighty cheese wheel down steep Cooper's Hill in Brockworth, near Gloucester, on May 31st 2010. The order came in March that year when the Gloucestershire police declared the event was too much of a health and safety risk because it was now attracting too many people. Inspector Stephen Norris said the organisers, the Cooper's Hill Cheese-Rolling Committee, had an obligation to ensure the safety of those attending and that the local police and county council had advised on how to create a safer event. He added that it was the cheese committee's decision to postpone the cheese chase that year. One of the committee's members, Richard Jefferies, admitted the decision was taken after police and council advice, adding: 'Last year 15,000 spectators tried to come to the event, by far the most we have ever seen and we just could not cope.' Mr Jefferies said he hoped the event would take place in 2011 in a revised form. But for some, the sense of danger and excitement is all part of the fun. Commented Robin Hammond of the Really Exciting Adventure Club: 'I do understand the issues about the crowd but wish that the local authorities had worked harder to ensure that we don't lose another part of our British culture to health and safety.'

7

No Laughing Matter

It was an email joke poking fun at the Irish, but BT bosses did not see the funny side and suspended thirty of its Leicester call centre workers in February 2009. Here is the joke in full:

Two Irishmen, Paddy and Gerry, drive to the top of the Connor Pass, where Gerry looks down at the 1,000ft drop and says 'Dis looks like a grand place.'

He takes two budgies out of a box, puts one on each shoulder and jumps off. Paddy watches the birds fly off and Gerry fall to the bottom, killing himself stone dead.

Looking down, Paddy shakes his head and says: 'Stuff dat. Dis budgie-jumping is too dangerous for me!' Moments later, Seamus arrives. He walks up to the edge of the cliff carrying another box and a shotgun. 'Hi Paddy, watch dis,' Seamus says. He lets a parrot out of the box, then throws himself over the edge of the cliff with the gun. Paddy watches as halfway down Seamus takes the gun and shoots the parrot.

Seamus carries on plummeting until he hits the bottom and breaks every bone. Paddy shakes his head and says, 'I'm never trying dat parrot-shooting either!'

Paddy is just getting over the shock when Sean appears. Sean pulls a chicken out, takes it by the legs and hurls himself off the cliff. He falls until he hits a rock and breaks his spine.

Once more Paddy shakes his head. 'Stuff dat, lads. First dere was Gerry budgie-jumping, den Seamus parrot-shooting and now Sean and his hen-gliding!'

Said one BT worker: 'The joke was sent around the office as a bit of fun. Everyone is worried about their jobs but we all try to cheer each other up. It was light-hearted but one person complained and suddenly managers were grilling people about the joke and saying it was offensive and could be interpreted as a racist slur on Irish people. I'm a quarter Irish and I didn't think it was offensive.'

But a BT spokesman said: 'A complaint was made about a joke which could be offensive to some people. BT takes these matters seriously and will investigate any allegations.'

A representative of the Leicester Irish Society was certainly not offended, saying: 'The Irish are famous for their sense of humour and it seems BT have lost theirs. The English and Irish communities have a history of taking the mickey out of each other. Suspending staff over a little joke is stupid. It would be funny if it wasn't so serious for the people whose jobs are on the line.' This attitude was backed up by the Communication Workers Union who said it was 'incredible' that BT could spend money on such 'a petty, meaningless investigation with customers very likely picking up the bill'.

March heralded the end of the Pantomime Dame – well, the camp ones anyway. For a new law was announced that would make it illegal to stereotype gay life – and that included our traditional Widow Twankey-type characters, and all similar entertainment on the radio and television as well as in books. In short, the Government wanted to push legislation through Parliament that would make it a serious crime to use any language which could be construed as offensive to gay men and women. But as gay celebrity Christopher Biggins announced: 'Showbiz, camp theatrics and dazzling wit helped to pave the way for gay rights. They should be cherished, not suppressed.

It is bitterly ironic that, in the name of tolerance, the Government is moving towards a culture of intolerance . . .'

Gender jokes caused other problems that month when it was revealed that fifty people had been invited to take part in a survey at a police liaison meeting in Wolverhampton. They were all handed electronic handsets and given their first instructions: 'Press A if you're male and B if you're female.' Someone asked what you would do if you were transgendered. Conservative councillor Jonathan Yardley replied with a smile: 'You could press A and B together.' Unfortunately for Mr Yardley, he was replying to a partner of a transgendered person – who was also at the meeting. The couple made a complaint to the police over 48-year-old Mr Yardley's 'homophobic' remark and he was summoned to meet with a police sergeant and inspector who criticised his sense of humour. 'They put me through the mill and asked me to confirm what I'd said and told me a complaint had been made and I could be prosecuted,' said Mr Yardley. 'I find it ridiculous you can get in trouble over an off-the-cuff remark. I didn't even know there was a transgender person there.' Mr Yardley, who did not face any charges, was unhappy that police time was wasted when he had been trying to get more police in his area to combat burglary and car crime. He added: 'I blame the Government for all the edicts they send out which seem to stop the police doing their real job and involve them in bureaucracy. Any innocuous remark now has to be investigated.' But said Chief Superintendent Richard Green, head of police in Wolverhampton West: 'At the time he (Mr Yardley) thanked the officers for discussing the matter with him and the appropriate and proportionate way they dealt with the matter.'

. . . The police had good reason to be sensitive over the transgender issue. Transgender serving and retired police officers and civilian staff unofficially formed the National Trans Police Association in 2008 to help with 'gender identity issues'. The group had the support of police forces. It went official in March

2010 when its 100 members made a bid for state funding while 'launching itself on the world' at the Bramshill police staff college in Hook, Hampshire. Chair of the association, Stephanie Robinson said: 'We are hoping that a few high-profile figures will be able to join us at the launch to help celebrate the achievement and what it means to be a transgender person in the 21st century.' There were some, of course, who questioned the need for any of it. John Midgley of the Campaign Against Political Correctness said: 'We don't need organisations like this. It's just madness.' Our good friend Matthew Elliott of the TaxPayers' Alliance had plenty to say. 'The police force should welcome people of every gender, sexuality, creed and race. However, they should be united in the fight against crime, not divided into competing political campaign groups. Even if people think it's productive to form cliques within the police, there is no way we should be diverting money from catching criminals.' This view was supported by Tory MP Philip Davies who shares the view of most of us. 'I don't care if a police officer is gay, straight, transgender or whatever. I just want them to catch criminals. If they get any funds out of tax-payers' income, that would be completely and utterly unacceptable. Everyone a few years ago said the police were institutionally racist. Now they are institutionally politically correct.'

Children have sung about Humpty Dumpty and his falling off a wall for years without suffering any trauma over his unhappy end. But in 2009 it was decided to change the nursery rhyme's ending from all the King's horses and all the King's men not being able to put Humpty together again, to 'made Humpty happy again . . .' The change was made for an October broadcast of the BBC children's programme *Something Special* aimed at children with learning difficulties, but also enjoyed by all pre-school children. The BBC insisted the change was made not to give the rhyme a cheerful ending in these politically correct times, but to be 'creative and entertaining'. But commented John Midgley of the Campaign Against Political Correctness: 'This is an unnecessary and outrageous piece of political correctness directed at young children. I very much doubt that any child has in the slightest bit been traumatised by Humpty Dumpty or any other age-old nursery rhyme.' In another children's programme, *Big Cook, Little Cook* which encourages little ones to learn to cook, the Little Miss Muffet rhyme was changed to her making friends with the spider who sat down beside her instead of being frightened away by it. Commented Tom Harris, Labour MP for Glasgow South: 'Kids should be exposed to real life a bit, not cosseted away. I think it's becoming a bit too much of a trend with the BBC. We need to stop this moronic activity.' When Enid Blyton's granddaughter, Sophie Smallwood wrote the first Noddy book in forty-six years she omitted one of the author's established and original characters. The book was published in October 2009 without Noddy's golliwog friend. Gollies had already been declared a racist invention some years previously. Said Ms Smallwood: 'I thought it would cause more upset to recreate something that had moved on . . .'

It was a case of 'pull the other one' – only in the case of the Christmas crackers joining the realms of political correctness, it was sadly true. Many jokes were axed from crackers because they were deemed unsuitable in these PC times. Taboo subjects included jokes about mothers-in-law, transvestites and 'cruel animal' jokes. The changes were announced in November 2009 by Swantex, Britain's biggest cracker-maker after it claimed research had shown traditional jokes were in need of an overhaul. Out went such old favourites as 'What is green and turns red at the push of a button?' – answer 'A frog in a liquidiser' and 'What do you call a drunk working at an upholstery shop? – answer 'A recovering alcoholic' and in came such gems as 'What do angry mice send each other at Christmas?' – answer 'Cross mouse cards.' A new cracker innovation was the introduction of 'conversation starters' – slips of paper with such questions as 'With whom would you least like to be stuck in a lift?' A spokesman for Swantex said all jokes are tested on a panel in laboratory conditions (i.e. over lunch with 'optional wine') and that jokes that fail to 'register a smile or a groan are not included in crackers'.

It was so heartening to hear in March 2009 that one man in particular was plainly fed up with the gobbledegook that has become Britain's 'official language'. That man was Richard Stokoe who compiled a list of 200 'council-speak' phrases that should be banned. He was a brave fellow indeed. For Mr Stokoe was actually working on behalf of the Local Government Association of which he is 'head of news'. He was tasked with converting the baffling bureaucratic balderdash into easy-to-understand English. Commented Mr Stokoe: 'Call me old-fashioned, but speaking plain English is the only way to get things started properly.' The Plain English Campaign warmly welcomed the list, adding that although it was not saying people 'are not intelligent enough or able enough to under-stand. It is the context in which the words are used that makes them gobbledegook.' One example which really riled Mr Stokoe was the phrase 'predictors of beaconicity'. He said he had no idea what it meant, even though it was the name of a 20-page report. Mr Stokoe, who first produced a list of 100 meaningless words in 2007, admitted the new list was designed to provoke controversy. He said: 'When I published the first list I had never seen such a strong response. It is dumbing down but those at the bottom of society cannot read very well and you have to make sure they can get access to services.' The Campaign Against Political Correctness (our kind of people!) said that while the list was well-meaning, it provided evidence that coun-cils had 'lost touch with reality'. Have they? Well, here is a sample of Mr Stokoe's banned words with what they really mean:

Across-the-piece: working together
Autonomous: independent
Best practice: best way

Blue-sky thinking: new ideas
Bottom-up: listening to people
Can-do culture: getting the job done
Citizen empowerment: people power
Core principles: beliefs
Coterminosity: all singing from the same hymn sheet (we would personally prefer 'all thinking the same'!)
Democratic legitimacy: voted in
Distorts spending priorities: ignores people's needs
Early win: success
Empowerment: people power
Flexibilities and freedoms: power to do the right thing
Functionality: use
Improvement levers: tools to get the job done
Interface: talking
Level playing field: equal
Lowlights: worst bits
Normalising: making normal
Outsourced: privatised
Parameter: limits
Place-shaping: providing places where people can thrive
Potentialities: chances
Rationalisation: cut
Risk-based: safest way
Seedbed: idea
Service users: people
Social exclusion: poverty
Tested for soundness: what works
Toolkit: guidance
Top-down: ignores people
Worklessness: unemployed

The list could go on and on – and indeed it does with such 'what the hell do they mean?' phrases as 'cohesive communities', 'holistic governance', 'peer challenge', 'predictors of beaconicity' and 'self-aggrandisement'.

Talking in a totally tortured way was the badge of the Noughties . . . and indeed will not go away easily. At the start of 2010, a new list of 'Office Waffle' was compiled by recruitment firm Office Angels with managing director David Clubb commenting: 'Trying to talk the talk isn't particularly productive and doesn't make you seem more professional. While this jargon is amusing, my advice would be that nothing beats plain talking.' Some of what has been described as the worst office gobbledegook for ten years included:

> We need the right pin number – this needs to work
> A lighthouse on a cloudy night – coming up with a bright idea
> Let's not try to build a chestnut fence to keep the sand dunes in – let's confront the problem head-on
> Funding streams – money
> Goldfish bowl-facilitated conversation – frank, round the table discussion
> I'm coming into this with an open kimono – I'm throwing the idea into the open
> Finger in the air figure – an estimate
> Expecting the moon on a stick – clients with demanding expectations
> I think someone needs a bite of the reality sandwich – they need to be more practical
> Wash-up session – meeting discussing current problems

One has always looked to the BBC for guidance on the Queen's English. But just like many others in these politically correct, positively crazy times, the Beeb was just as guilty in the gobbledegook ratings. One minute it announced it was shedding its silly job titles to keep licence-payers sweet; the next, it was advertising a very confusing vacancy indeed. In November 2009 the BBC came under fire for creating such job titles as Solutions Architect, Organisational Development and Change Director, Director of Audiences and a Reward Director (with the very rewarding annual salary of £196,000). Even a top employee, one Simon Nelson, admitted his title BBC Vision Controller of Multi-Platform and Portfolio, was 'completely barmy'. In January 2010, the BBC advertised for a Change Lead, the successful candidate being 'responsible for shaping and managing the execution of the change ambition' for the Digital Media Initiative Programme and responsible too, for ensuring the Change Strategy is 'operating implementable and effective' AND with 'visibility of all change initiatives' AND responsible for 'driving decisions'. Conservative culture spokesman Jeremy Hunt said he was sure most BBC staff would wonder what a 'Change Lead' was and why it warranted a suggested six-figure salary. A BBC spokesman explained: 'Change Lead is an accepted and clearly identifiable job title in any organisation where the way people work is changing. In this case the BBC is seeking to fill this temporary position with a senior manager with broad and extensive knowledge of implementing change programmes in large and complex organisations to successfully deliver a change programme as part of the Digital Media Initiative.'

Not long afterwards, the BBC declared it was definitely going to ban its barmy job titles because they didn't really inform the public what people in the jobs actually did. Said a BBC source: 'The corporation is trying to become more transparent and has recognised that the public needs to recognise what people do.' The BBC said it would change existing meaningless titles to ones that made sense and ensure all senior management jobs would have to pass a 'clarity and commonsense' test when advertised.

. . . That lifted our hearts – until later that month, March 2010, we heard that the good old Beeb had been funding two-day workshops for its staff to learn how to use that great (and free to sign up with) social network Facebook (as well as Twitter and Bebo). The BBC had run sixty-nine 'Making The Web Work For You' sessions since their launch in November 2009, with 476 staff members taking part. But even some BBC staff felt uncomfortable about the classes. Said one: 'We're meant to be belt-tightening. It is an astonishing waste of money. Teenagers who can barely read or write have managed to teach themselves.' Others pointed out that many of the staff already knew how to use the sites. Conservative MP Philip Davies, on Parliament's Culture, Media and Sports select committee said: 'It's just an absolute waste of money. It is ridiculous. These are the actions of an organisation that has so much money it does not know what to do with it.' Unlike many private sector employers, the BBC does not restrict its workers' use of social networking sites. It said the two-day courses cost 'less than £50' a person – which still added up to nearly £24,000. Justifying the web courses, a BBC spokesman said they helped journalists 'develop effective and comprehensive internet research and social media skills' and that most of the cost was covered by 'fixed resource', adding: 'The aim is to help journalists find original stories, case studies and pictures using the latest web techniques. It is not about how to set up a Facebook account.'

It wasn't just the BBC coming under fire for failing to less than impress the public at the start of 2010, with the news that of 890 programmes shown by a Welsh-language TV channel funded with nearly £1million of public money, during three weeks in February and March 196 had the grand viewing figures of, errh, officially no-one. The channel, S4C, the Channel 4 of Wales, recorded zero viewers. Well, to be fair, a few people had tuned in but the figure of 1,000 was too low to be officially registered. Just 139 out of all the station's entire programmes for that period were watched by more than 10,000 viewers. Programmes which lacked pulling power included a children's cartoon called *Sali Mali and Tocyn* in which presenters visit Celtic countries and regions, and a soccer show called *Sgorio* which scored an own goal with a zero-viewing rating when it screened highlights of European football. Sgorio, incidentally, is Welsh for 'score'. Commented former Conservative Welsh Office Minister Rod Richards, a Welsh speaker and broadcaster: 'I am disappointed and saddened by these figures. It is shocking that so many of

S4C's programmes do not seem to resonate with the public, and worrying for anyone concerned about the Welsh language. S4C gets a huge amount of public money and it's time it was dragged into the 21st century, kicking and screaming if necessary.' Things were so dire that Mr Richards called for the BBC to be given back responsibility for Welsh-language TV in Wales; a responsibility it had before Cardiff-based S4C was set up in 1982 when Channel 4 was launched. The TaxPayers' Alliance summed up what everyone was thinking, that 'these figures make clear that S4C is a huge waste of tax-payers' money'. Chief Executive Matthew Elliott added: 'It seems that even Welsh speakers aren't interested in its output, which is a dismal failure. The whole public sector has got to make big cuts to balance the books and a TV channel no-one watches is something that should be first on the list to scrap.'

8

Keeping Up Appearances

It was a case of the road being paved with good intentions – but also an over-the-top desire to curb street names causing offence. In January Lewes District Council in East Sussex drew up a list of guidelines to avoid new road signs being sniggered at for suggested double entendres. The council said that 'names capable of deliberate misinterpretation such as Hoare Road, Typple Avenue and Corfe Close (4 Corfe Close) etc' should be banned. So too were 'aesthetically unsuitable names' such as Gaswork Road and Coalpit Lane. Also in the guidelines were street names 'which could give offence and names which encourage defacing name plates'. The council was no doubt frustrated that it could do little about existing names such as Juggs Road and Cockshut Road. Former councillor and resident of Cockshut Road, Rachel Powell, said: 'I would hate for the name to change. It has some history. I can see with political correctness why the council would not want these sort of names but it is a pity.'

It seemed the perfect 'welcome home' gesture: flying the English national flag from the roof to greet new Coldstream Guards, twins 18-year-old Richard and Robert Smithson. But proud father Robert Smithson was thwarted when someone complained. An official from Sunderland City Council wrote to 42-year-old Mr Smithson threatening him with a fine of up to £2,500 for illegally flying the flag from his home. Further, he was breaking planning rules by flying the Cross of St George at the wrong angle – because it was horizontal and not vertical it was classed as a form of advertising and required a licence from the local authority. 'I would have laughed had the whole thing not been so serious. It was ridiculous,' said Mr Smithson. 'For someone to put in a complaint about the national flag is bad enough, but the way the council has handled it is appalling.' It turned out that the council had misinterpreted their own rules and that national flags were specifically excluded from its advertising regulations. Phil Barrett, glorying under the title of Director of Development and Regeneration said the council decided the flag could stay. 'We will be writing to Mr Smithson and apologising for any upset,' he said.

It took Tony Pye three months to decorate England's best cockle and whelk stall and then he was left shell-shocked by a council ruling that said he had to put it back just the way it was.

Tony's crime? He fixed seashells to his stall in Folkestone, Kent, in the belief that the decoration would add to the ambience of the seaside setting. Officials at Shepway District Council disagreed, saying the shells were not in keeping with the seaside location. They ordered 57-year-old Mr Pye to restore his stall back to its black-stained weatherboarding on his award-winning harbour pitch because they said that appearance was more 'sympathetic' to the appearance of the area rather than shells.

Mr Pye, who has had the stall for twenty years, was quite rightly angry that all his efforts to brighten it up for the summer season were for all nothing after the council came down on him in February 2009. He said: 'I spent days collecting the shells and gluing them onto the kiosk. Everyone comments on how good the seashells look as opposed to the depressing boards. I hoped the new design would help attract customers. To be told I have to take all the shells off now after all my hard work is depressing to say the least.'

Locals supported Mr Pye, whose kiosk has been awarded the title of Best Seafish Stall in England by the English Heritage group. Said resident, 38-year-old Alan Parkinson: 'Tony has spent a lot of effort in the freezing cold putting these shells on his stall. All he's doing is trying to get more customers and make a living. It's a disgrace that the council are now telling him he has to remove them all.' Another local, 21-year-old Rebecca Scott added: 'I've watched Tony hard at work and he's transformed it from a dull black building to something magical.'

Shepway District Council said Mr Pye needed planning permission for his decorative work. 'The building is in a conservation area and the council has a duty to ensure that any works that need planning permission either preserve or enhance this. The shell cladding needs planning permission and officers believe it detracts from the appearance of the harbour.'

The last word comes from Folkestone road-sweeper, 28-year-old Gavin Hunt who commented: 'It's ridiculous. I don't know what it's got to do with the planners. They're a bunch of nosey-parkers who make people's lives a misery.'

In April, 28-year-old artist Anton Cataldo was desperate to track down two of his paintings that had gone missing after he had placed them on the roof of his car and unthinkingly driven off. In an attempt to recover the paintings – portraits of his parents' Labradors Oscar and Sam – Mr Cataldo made posters of the pictures, included his phone number, added a £100 reward and stapled them to twelve trees in his local park in Brighton.

Mr Cataldo did get a response to his plea, but it was not the news he had been hoping for. An enforcement officer of Brighton and Hove City Council contacted him to say he was harming 'living' trees and fined the artist £75 for 'wounding the bark of a tree in any way that can lead to attack by airborne fungal spores which in the worst case scenario, could lead to the loss of the tree'. The email to Mr Cataldo added that although the council 'genuinely hope' his paintings were returned, it 'simply cannot allow every person who loses property to resort to the kind of actions as taken by yourself'. Mr Cataldo said he found the email patronising and said that although not an expert, he doubted very much that a staple could cause 'so much damage to a tree it would actually die'. He complained about the fine and it was later cancelled with a council spokesman admitting: 'This was probably a case of an officer who was a little bit over-zealous.'

No-one likes litter louts. But then who could honestly believe someone would drop money on the streets to cause offence? Well, two police officers of the Strathclyde force for a start. For when arthritis sufferer Stewart Smith, 36, accidentally let a £10 note flutter from his hand as he left a charity shop, the two officers first pointed out the matter – and then accused him of littering. They then issued Mr Smith with a £50 fixed-penalty notice.

One can only assume the police were enforcing their zero tolerance to litter in the Scottish town of Ayr in June. Said Mr Smith, who has been forced to give up work because of his illness and who had bought a T-shirt at the shop: 'I came out of the shop with my T-shirt under my arm. I put £7 in coins into my front pocket as I was going to buy some juice. I thought I was putting a £10 note and the receipt in my back pocket. But my shirt was hanging over the pocket and the £10 note, along with the receipt, fell onto the street.' After having his 'crime' pointed out to him, Mr Smith tried to explain it was an honest mistake. A spokesman for Strathclyde Police insisted Mr Smith had dropped several papers and had ignored a warning to pick them up – though the fixed-penalty notice read: 'You did drop a price ticket' and said: 'An individual was seen throwing papers on the street. When he was approached and spoken to about it, he recovered the money he had thrown away but repeated his actions with the papers. He was therefore ticketed.' But commented Scottish Tory justice spokesman Bill Aitken: 'Clearly no-one is going to throw away a £10 note. From what he says it would seem fairly clear that he (Mr Smith) dropped both items by mistake.' Added Conservative MP Philip Davies: 'This seems on the face of it to be a very petty action. This sounds like a case where common sense has been ignored.'

Young mum 26-year-old Laura Whotton was told to stop breast-feeding her baby because she was contravening a leisure centre's poolside food and drink ban. Mrs Whotton was feeding 3-month-old Joshua while also trying to keep an eye on her other son, 4-year-old Thomas who was playing in the toddlers' pool. A male lifeguard approached her and told her she could not breast-feed in public because there were children present. He offered Mrs Whotton a 'private room' but she refused as it meant leaving little Thomas. Mrs Whotton left the John Carroll Leisure Centre in Nottingham when she realised the lifeguard was not going to back down. She said: 'I felt really angry at being treated like that. I wasn't embarrassed because I didn't have anything on show. People in bikinis were showing more skin and breast than me. It's the most natural thing in the world and I was made to feel like I was doing something terrible.' Mrs Whotton wrote and complained to Nottingham City Council who answered that it was local policy to allow mothers to breast-feed in all council centres including leisure centres. The only exception to this rule is in a swimming pool and surrounding area where there is a policy of 'no food and drink' in the interests of safety and hygiene. It added: 'This rule also covers breast-feeding, as it would the bottle-feeding of a baby.' But the council later gave Mrs Whotton a 'full and open apology' and agreed to review its policy.

It seemed like an excellent hard-hitting campaign at the time – posters showing the effect that years in prison would have on two gangland murderers. The move was aimed at discouraging violence and gun crime. But the Greater Manchester police force faced a court action by families of the two thugs who said the poster was an infringement of human rights and had led to 'increasing hostility' from the public. Civil rights group Liberty also said the poster infringed Article 8 of the European Convention on Human Rights which provides a right to respect for one's 'private and family life and home'.

The poster, pasted up on billboards in Manchester in June, pictured gang leaders and convicted murderers 29-year-old Colin Joyce and 33-year-old Lee Amos, at their current age and how they would look upon release in 2048 and 2044 respectively. But said James Welch, spokesman for Liberty: 'This case is not about protecting convicted criminals behind bars but about safeguarding innocent family members who have done nothing wrong. The police should be keeping the peace, not stirring up trouble. Liberty will always protect vulnerable people no matter how unfortunate their family relationships.'

Commented Chief Constable Peter Fahy: 'We are in the business of saving lives and will do all we can to prevent young people falling victim to gun crime and gang life. These were among the most dangerous men in Manchester and our communities are safer with them locked up. Before the campaign we consulted with the Home Office and campaigners who have been on the front line of the battle against gun crime – and the families of the victims. All of them supported us. We believed it was the right thing to do – and we still do.' After the imprisonment of Joyce and Amos the number of gang-related incidents in Manchester's notorious Moss Side area was reduced by 92 per cent.

When Di Pitchford tragically lost her 17-year-old son Gary in a car crash, she was touched that his friends raised £137 for a memorial bench to be placed alongside his grave in a council cemetery. But Colchester Borough Council did not approve of the tribute, demanding that it be replaced with an authorised bench costing almost £700. In July Councillor Tim Young, with responsibility for the cemetery, said benches had to be of a special hardwood and long-lasting, adding: 'We do not want anybody just to buy a bench for £30 that will bring down the standard and quality.' Mrs Pitchford, 43, and her family were also told the bench was 'disturbing mourners' at the cemetery. She said: 'I was disgusted. I feel someone is being a real jobsworth. They have obviously never lost a child. . . . In my opinion our bench is sturdier and better quality than the council's one. I think they are preying on grieving families and charging them extortionate prices.'

He was always a favourite with schoolchildren who grew up with their comic hero and loved his mischievous antics. But today, the Dennis the Menace cartoon character has been transformed into something, well, less menacing. Originating in the *Beano* comic in 1951, Dennis was given a new image for a BBC children's television series in August. He still wore his trademark black and red shirt and black shorts, but his beady eyes and sneer were replaced with rounder eyes and a jolly smile. He also had to drop, quite literally, his catapult, his 'wanton destruction' and his habit of tormenting Walter the Softy in case it was seen as assault on homosexuals. The good news for Dennis was that he would no longer be hit on the bottom with a slipper by his father. Said a BBC spokesman: 'Dennis can't be seen to use weapons and giving other kids grief in a BBC cartoon.' Dennis's fellow rogue Gnasher had his personality changed too, and was banned from taking bites out of other characters – a trait of his from the good old days. Long-term Dennis the Menace fan, 64-year-old Jim Stewart commented: 'It's ridiculous. Dennis is supposed to be a little bit edgy.'

The red and white barber's shop pole had stood outside Rob Grice's shop in Wigan for nineteen years and had never caused anyone to complain – or indeed caused anyone any harm. But then one day it was declared a threat to the health and safety of passing pedestrians and snatched away by the council. The reasons, declared the council, were because 'we work closely with access groups and it is our duty to look after the interests of people in wheelchairs and with white sticks. Objects like these are not as stable as fixed street signs and we are being encouraged by Government to be much more proactive over things like this . . . the shop is in a narrow street. It was an accident waiting to happen. The proprietor was issued with a warning but he failed to respond so we were obliged to take it off him.' Mr Grice was, however, told he could have his pole back if he paid the council £100. The 38-year-old barber quite rightly felt like pulling his hair out and said: 'Nobody has tripped over the pole in the nineteen years I've owned the shop. There are bins and lampposts along the street but they are not considered safety hazards. The pole let our customers know when we were open and now it has been taken away.'

In October, villagers of Aldbourne, near Malmesbury in Wiltshire, faced court action after putting up a flashing sign requesting motorists to slow down. It seemed to work as in just one week around 2,680 motorists on the B4192 were clocked by the £2,800 warning sign for going over 33mph in the 30mph area. Some were even driving as fast as 60mph. But Wiltshire Council did not take kindly to what they said was an unauthorised sign, saying it broke planning laws and 'if speed signs are in the wrong place they can cause accidents . . .' One resident, 73-year-old Michael Edmonds who helped with the purchase of the sign, commented: 'It's laughable. We are the ones trying to uphold the law . . . and are being treated like criminals . . .'

Grieving widower, 77-year-old retired factory worker Stanley Brown found comfort in laying bunches of flowers on his wife's grave. But his touching gesture was restricted by the health and safety police who said only one bunch at a time could be placed on the grave of his wife Violet, at Gorstage Cemetery, in Weaverham, near Northwich, Cheshire. One £20 bunch of flowers was removed and put in a shed. Then Mr Brown received a letter saying he had broken the cemetery rules because too many flowers caused an obstruction to gardeners cutting the grass and they might fall over. Mr Brown was naturally very upset, saying: 'If I lay flowers, one of my children or grandchildren who wants to pay their respects and lay flowers for their mum and grandma can't because it's against the rules. It's disgusting that when I put flowers on the grave no-one else in my family can because of these jobsworth rules.' Said cemetery committee chairman John Freeman: 'Plot owners are only allowed room for a single set of flowers due to the layout and upkeep of the cemetery.'

Most want to wear their poppy with pride in memory of those who lost their lives in the two world wars. But even this touching tradition was not exempt from controversy in 2009. First of all poppy-sellers from the Royal British Legion were banned from shaking their collection tins in case they were seen as a 'public nuisance'. Then staff at the forty-eight libraries in Derbyshire were told they could not have collection tins and boxes because it would mean they were supporting 'particular charities at the expense of others'. They were told to remove the tins and boxes 'immediately' in emails sent by Derbyshire County Council's Operations Department. Operations Manager Ann Ainsworth wrote: 'I need to reinforce that the County Council does not support specific charities and does not provide opportunities for any charities to collect donations via Derbyshire Libraries . . . clearly this also excludes collection boxes for the Royal British Legion Poppy Appeal. Please ensure collection boxes have not been accepted for public display during this year's appeal in any of our buildings.' The dictate caused so much upset that the council later backed down, with council leader Andrew Lewer saying: 'We are wholeheartedly supporters of the Armed Forces and I am very happy for libraries to sell poppies on behalf of the British Legion. To avoid confusion about past policies, I will be letting all libraries know they can sell poppies this year.'

When grandfather and residents' group chairman Thomas Catcheside, 67, fell into dispute with Cambridge Council in October over what he felt was the slippery conditions of communal steps at his block of flats, he found himself being treated like a very slippery customer by the police – and was arrested in a terrifying dawn raid and held in a cell for six hours.

He also had his fingerprints and a DNA sample taken. Mr Catcheside's 'crime' was to use the 'F-word' to a council official who was visiting him about his dangerous stairs complaint which had dragged on for three years. He lost his temper when the official would not let him listen to a telephone call to his supervisor and shouted: 'Don't you tell me what I can and can't do in my own ****ing place.' The official complained he had felt 'threatened' and six days later Mr Catcheside was at the centre of the dawn raid as he slept in bed with his 62-year-old wife, Deborah. He was ordered to change and was then driven off in a police van. He was accused of 'causing harassment, alarm or distress in a public place' – even though, of course, he had been in his own home at the time of the bad language. During his time in the cell, the retired lorry driver who suffers from asthma and high blood pressure suffered a panic attack and had to be seen by a police doctor. He was only allowed to leave after being given an £80 fixed-penalty notice. Describing his ordeal, Mr Catcheside said: 'My wife and I were asleep when the police arrived. I opened the door and they just barged in. I told them to wait a minute but they followed me into my bedroom where my wife was in bed. She was so embarrassed she hid behind a cushion. I was frightened and angry as I felt like I was being criminalised. It was so heavy-handed. The police seem to have trouble catching proper criminals and here they were dragging me down to the station for defending my rights. I admit I swore, but I was frustrated because we have been fighting to get these stairs improved for years, writing letter after letter, and the council has taken no notice.' A spokesman for Cambridgeshire police said they had been following 'national policy' and responding to reports of an assault 'which is a serious offence. The suspect was arrested at the earliest possible opportunity, which happened to be at 5.35am.' It was later decided there was not enough evidence to charge Mr Catcheside with assault but his admission of being abusive resulted in the fine and 'words of advice about his behaviour'. Robert Hollingsworth of City Homes, a housing association which runs council housing for

Cambridge council, said they had reported the incident to the police because their representative had felt 'threatened'.

The Greater Manchester Police force was not impressed with the man they had chosen to train special constables and dismissed him. Not because 62-year-old Alan Power was bad at his job – but because he believes messages from the dead can help solve criminal investigations. But Mr Power, who has attended a spiritualist church for twenty-nine years won through at an Employment Appeal Tribunal hearing which, despite an appeal by the Greater Manchester Police Authority, ruled that spiritualism qualified as a 'religious or philosophical belief'. Judge Peter Clark agreed with Judge Pete Russell's earlier decision that 'in common with other spiritualists, the claimant believes in the existence of a God, that there is life after death and that the dead can be contacted through mediums', adding: 'There is no suggestion that the claimant does not genuinely believe in the tenets of faith.' It all left the way clear for Mr Power to bring a religious discrimination claim and he said: 'I haven't claimed costs and I'm not claiming compensation. It's about hurt feelings. I expect my religion to be respected.' Acting for the police, QC Mark Hill said the decision could open the gates for more unorthodox religions and quoted a 'Jedi Knights' defence – a reference to a co-ordinated campaign in the 2001 census when 390,000 people claimed to follow the religion from the *Star Wars* films.

Oh, the town centre Christmas tree, with its smell of pine and brightly-coloured decorations. Or not. Well, not in Poole, Dorset, anyway. Its Town Centre Management Board, comprising local businesses and organisations, decided in December 2009 that a 30ft tall traditional tree in the centre's Falkland Square was a danger to the public because it might topple over in high winds. So it was replaced by something resembling a giant green 33ft-high traffic cone, lit up at night and containing loudspeakers belting out Christmas carols but without decorations, or indeed branches. A traditional tree – the kind the town had enjoyed for the last twenty-five years or so – would have cost £500, plus £3,500 to decorate it using a 'cherry-picker'. The green cone in all its naked glory cost £14,000. Supporting the board's decision, town centre manager Richard Randall-Jones said: 'People think you can just go into the woods, chop down a tree and put it in the high street. But if it blows over and kills someone then we are liable for it. We are a coastal town and so we have strict health and safety guidelines around making the Christmas tree safe due to the high winds we suffer. We have to have guy ropes and hoardings to stop it falling over and hitting somebody.' Shoppers, however, were quite rightly not impressed. Said one: 'It looks like something that has just landed out of space. It looks nothing like a Christmas tree.' Commented another: 'At night it looks OK because it has lights on but it just looks weird during the day. A Christmas tree is a tree that looks nice on the eye and sways in the wind and smells nice when you go past it. This just looks odd.' There was also the suggestion that the extra £10,000 the massive 'fir cone' cost could have been better spent on public services. The Town Centre Management Board, however, stood as firm as their newly-introduced Christmas tree substitute. Added Mr Richard Randall-Jones: 'Children can walk right up to it and touch it and have their picture taken next to it. It looks pretty at night with the lights on. I challenge anyone who can find a better tree in the area.' A few days later, it was reported that the traffic cone tree was being replaced by a more traditional one after it was wrecked by protestors, was threatened to be burned to the ground and was the subject of a Facebook campaign involving more than 4,000 angry residents. Said one opposer: 'How did they think they would get away with a cone with fake turf on it? Either have a proper tree or don't have one at all.'

Hansel and Gretel, the original Brothers Grimm version: their evil mother persuades their father to abandon them in a forest because there is not enough food for them all. They find a gingerbread house and start to eat it because they are hungry. The house's owner, a witch, lures them inside and threatens to eat Hansel. Gretel manages to push the witch into an oven. The two children get home safely to a happy father who informs them their horrible mum is dead. Hansel and Gretel 2009: the two children are 'hoodie' yobs who steal the purse of their 'under the watchful eye of Social Services' mother (with Gretel threatening to break her brother's neck if he tells 'I pinched her pension'), mount a raid on a gingerbread house and intimidate the elderly occupant. The two bad children are arrested and sent to prison for criminal damage. They are only allowed out if they agree to be nice. That was the panto version at Keresley Newland Primary School in Coventry, Warwickshire. Some parents threatened to boycott the production with one commenting: 'It's a travesty that a jolly panto story has been changed into a bleak portrayal of modern Britain which is run by thugs.' Another said: 'The story has been totally butchered to drive home a message of bullying. It's an absolute disgrace and the writers have, frankly, killed the spirit of Christmas.' The modern version of Hansel and Gretel was partly funded by the charity Warwickshire Crimebeat and adapted by one of the school's teachers. Staff argued that it dealt with the issues of bullying, anti-social behaviour and that it taught children to respect other people's belongings. Panto director, teacher Rachel Cooper said: 'The play is a great opportunity for the community to get involved with our school and to remind people that bullying will not be tolerated.'

A hoodie of another kind encountered the thought police that same month when pensioner and great-grandmother 84-year-old Mrs Peggy Harden was asked to drop her fur-trimmed anorak hood as she walked through the Grand Arcade shopping mall in Cambridge. The order, from a security guard, was in line with the centre's 'no hoodie' policy in a bid to ban a somewhat younger and more unruly element. It is no wonder that 5ft 2in tall, arthritis sufferer Mrs Harden, who uses a walking stick and was accompanied by her 84-year-old husband Desmond, failed to see how she fitted into that category. She said after the incident – which left her feeling confused and intimidated – 'The arcade was cold and draughty inside but I was going to take my hood off before I went to the shops. The man started to approach me and he wore a uniform and a badge so I thought I'd done something wrong. I looked at him in amazement and he said something about security. I have to keep my head down when I walk because I can't see very well and I didn't really know what was happening.' A spokesman for the Grand Arcade later apologised to the couple but insisted: 'It's more about health and safety than intimidation. Grand Arcade has a "no-hood" policy to ensure a safe and enjoyable shopping experience for everyone. However, it is not our intention to cause any upset and we apologise for any stress this may have caused.' Peggy's husband was still less than pleased, saying: 'Older people with walking sticks aren't going to start hitting people. We felt a bit victimised, like we were being treated like criminals.' And the couple's daughter, 60-year-old Val Bennett added: 'If you could see them walking with their sticks you'd never think they were dangerous. If one falls over, the other goes too. When my mother told me I was incensed. There were plenty of young men walking around in hoodies, but the security guard was probably worried he would get a bop in the chops if he challenged any of them.'

Every school wants to appear on good form when it comes to its pupils' regular attendance. But in January, one school's determination to beat truancy was deemed by some as in a politically incorrect class of its own. Mrs Paula Sergeant, head teacher of Patcham High School in Brighton, East Sussex, came up with the idea of offering parents free flying lessons, High Street shop and spa salon vouchers if they managed to get their children not to miss a day's schooling each month. The names would then be put into a prize draw. The children were encouraged too, with an 'attendance raffle' in which they stood the chance of winning iPods and food treats if they accumulated enough attendance points. The school had recently been named in the 'top' 200 most improved schools in the country but still had the second-worst truancy rates. Justifying the idea, Mrs Sergeant said: 'Sometimes parents have a difficult time getting their kids into school so this is just another thing to try and help improve our attendances. We still have a long way to go and we need more of our children making an effort to come to school on a regular basis. There has been improvement but the pace of improvement has not been as fast as we would like so we are putting lots of things in place and we are particularly pushing this term.'

The approach to encouraging children's regular attendance in lessons was seen as bad form by critics though. Parents lobby group founder Margaret Morrissey said: 'It is surely a sad state of affairs where parents have to be bribed to comply with their legal duty and get their children to come to school and with something as expensive as flying lessons. The prizes will take a substantial amount of the school budget which could be spent on sensible things like books.' A spokesman for Brighton and Hove City Council supported the idea, however, saying: 'All schools are under pressure to improve attendance. Often rewards alongside sanctions for both parents and pupils can be very effective. The council supports schools to do everything they can to encourage children to attend and parents to take responsibility for ensuring they attend.' None of this impressed Conservative MP Graham Stuart, a member of the Commons Education Select Committee who thundered: 'What next? Will parents demand a rally-driving course or a drive in a Ferrari before they do their legal duty and send their children to be educated at school? You will end up letting parents think they can demand some sort of reward for simply doing what they should do as a matter of course. It is tantamount to child abuse not to make sure your children go to school. Without education no child has a chance of competing in the world and being able to make a decent, honest living.'

*   *   *

Can you do too much of a good job when it comes to cleaning up rubbish? Thurrock Council in Essex seemed to think you can. For when a group of seventeen volunteers from North Stifford Community Group spent three hours' hard work filling no less than forty-three bags with rubbish from the local streets and pavements, they were told their efforts were 'excessive'. That was because the three-man dustbin team who arrived on their rounds did the right thing and collected all the bags. Errh, but unfortunately, their van was so full they could not complete their rounds. It was all a bit of a mess, especially as it was the council who approved the 'operation bagful' and even provided the bin bags and litter-picking sticks. Out went an email from the council's cleaning manager, Ashley Cobett, who said: 'Please bear in mind that the weekend teams have their regular work to do borough-wide and forty-three bags and a sofa are a little excessive to collect. As this had filled up one of the vans they were unable to complete all of their work that day. I am happy to help voluntary organisations, but I would be very grateful if you would consider this for the future.' The volunteers had undertaken their clean-up following a petition signed by 300 villagers complaining about litter. Said Community Group vice-chairman, Gordon Roberts: 'The council's whole attitude to all this is crazy. They provided us with the bin bags and sticks to collect the rubbish in the first place. Then for them to turn round when a group of volunteers has spent hours helping tidy the village and say we have collected an excessive amount is total madness.' The clean-up was part of Keep Britain Tidy's 'Big Tidy Up' campaign and added Mr Roberts: 'It was a very successful day and the reality is that we pay our council tax and if the rubbish collectors did their job in the first place, we wouldn't even have to be there. We are a close-knit village and many members of the community who wanted this done are infuriated by the whole ridiculous situation.' A council spokesman later said the group had done an excellent job and apologised that the email was sent 'in error . . .'

*   *   *

Ex-councillor and grandfather, 84-year-old Graham Powell confronted a gang of youths who had been terrorising him and his 74-year-old wife Sybil for months. He ended up being arrested and charged with assault. The Powells had virtually been prisoners in their flat in Caldicot, near Newport, south Wales, after suffering four months of harassment by up to ten local youths aged between 11 and 15, who smashed their car lights, let down tyres, cut the car seat belts and poured flour and tomato sauce on the car bonnet. Mrs Powell had also twice been trapped in her garage by youths who had jammed the door shut and the couple had members of the gang peering through their window and ringing the doorbell of their home where they had hitherto lived happily for thirty-one years. The former leader of Gwent County Council eventually went to talk to the gang, one of whom claimed he hit him with his walking stick. According to Mr Powell this was not true and the youth had punched him and hurled two metal plant pots at him. He, however, was the one taken to a police station where he was kept for six hours and interrogated. He said: 'I remonstrated with the youth after my wife caught him fiddling with one of the letterboxes. He told me to mind my own XXXXXXX business and punched me on the arm. I poked my walking stick through the rails to stop him and he forced the stick down with his arm. I was amazed when police accused me of assault.' Mr Powell wrote a letter of complaint to the Gwent Chief Constable urging him to protect law-abiding citizens. A Gwent police spokesman confirmed an investigation into assault was taking place. Calling his tormentors 'feral' youths because they were wild and out of control, Mr Powell added: 'It's outrageous that instead of them being arrested I am facing standing in the dock.'

Young mum Kirsty Allen, 29, was fined £50 by a North-East Lincolnshire Council warden in Grimsby after her baby, 16-month-old Lennon, dropped a piece of banana out of his pram after falling asleep mid-munch. Although Kirsty saw the morsel drop, she did not feel compelled to retrieve it from the pavement as it fell into a puddle and was more than likely to be eaten by a bird or just rot away to nothing. The watching warden did not share the same opinion and handed Kirsty a £50 on-the-spot fine for littering. Said the irate mum: 'Lennon loves bananas and I had given him one to eat to settle him down. He must have finished eating it and left the end of it on the blanket. It rolled off the side of the pram and landed in a big puddle. I didn't really think of it as litter as I thought it would be eaten by birds or just decompose. The warden pulled me up and issued me with a £50 fine. I think it is disgusting. I was lost for words and trust me, that doesn't happen often.' Defending its action, 'interim environmental enforcement manager' John Wade said: 'It is standard procedure to issue a fixed-penalty notice to anybody who is caught littering. The offence was acknowledged by Mrs Allen and the council's community warden spoke to her about the consequences of waste being discarded. The stance of zero tolerance fines for littering will continue in a bid to improve public confidence and restore pride to our communities.'

The loony approach to littering (what do you think of it so far? Rubbish!) was further highlighted in February 2010 when the Sawbridgeworth Evening Women's Institute in Hertfordshire was threatened with £80 fines for handing out flyers for a charity art exhibition. Retired medical secretary and grandmother, 68-year-old Liz Day and three fellow WI ladies were warned by a council litter warden (remember we have those now!) that it was illegal to hand out the flyers which could end up on the floor and be classified as litter, particularly if the fliers were tucked under car windscreen wipers. The women were also told they needed a licence to hand out the adverts. It was so lucky for the ladies that the council litter warden let them off with a warning 'because he was in a good mood'. Mrs Day, the WI group president, was left both bemused and bothered by the incident. She said the women had felt 'criminalised' and added: 'We had no idea handing out a flyer to someone could be illegal.

You see people doing it all the time. We were shocked and very upset because this is for charity. This is the first time in six years someone has told us we must not hand out our flyers. We went and regrouped. But we had to stop because we didn't want to be fined. None of us knew it was illegal, but who does know?' After a discussion among themselves, the WI members gave their flyers to stallholders at the Sawbridge Farmers' Market who are allowed to hand out leaflets to customers. A local council spokesman said that its Area Environmental Inspectors (litter wardens to you and me) had intervened to advise the ladies that putting leaflets on car windscreens was illegal. He said: 'Unfortunately when leaflets are left on people's cars the tendency is to throw them on the floor, which causes a litter issue.' The women say they were not putting their flyers on cars and are not happy that next time they undertake their charity leaflet distribution they will have to apply for a licence. Added Mrs Day: 'It's such a shame. This is all just more red tape. I know these people have a job to do but this was over the top. We enjoy doing this every year but being threatened with a fine doesn't really make it worth the hassle.' The annual art exhibition raises money for good causes, one year raising £500 for an air ambulance. Our good friend Mark Wallace, campaign director of the TaxPayers' Alliance felt the council's reaction was a rubbish approach to people trying to do something for the community, saying it was 'draconian and completely over the top' adding: 'These ladies were doing something for charity in their own time at their own expense. If anything, the council should be encouraging them, not issuing ridiculous threats.'